ve **Better** and **Longer**

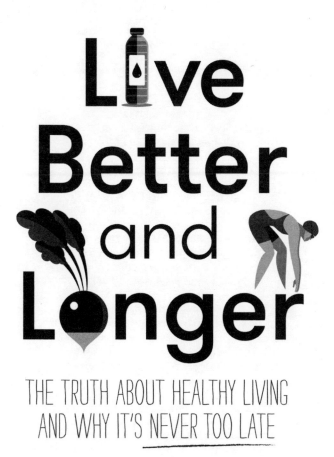

Live Better and Longer

THE TRUTH ABOUT HEALTHY LIVING AND WHY IT'S NEVER TOO LATE

MICHEL CYMES

With the collaboration of Patrice Romedenne
Translated from the French by Sam Alexander

Quercus

First published in France in 2016 by Editions Stock under the title
Vivez Mieux et Plus Longtemps

This edition first published in Great Britain in 2017 by

Quercus Editions Ltd
Carmelite House
50 Victoria Embankment
London EC4Y 0DZ

An Hachette UK company

A CIP catalogue record for this book is available
from the British Library

TPB ISBN 978 1 78648 293 8
EBOOK ISBN 978 1 78648 294 5

Printed a   d bound in Great   'lc.

Contents

Introduction

I once came across a quote that said something like: 'The poorest of the poor wouldn't swap their health for all the money in the world, but the richest of the rich would gladly give up their piles of cash to be healthy again.' I think that's pretty much spot on. It goes to show that our health is a gift of immeasurable value. It is, to pinch a nice line attributed to Edme-Pierre Chauvot de Beauchêne (physician to Charles X) 'the most precious of treasures, the easiest to lose and, paradoxically, the least well protected'.

No one escapes their genetic heritage. No one escapes their upbringing either. But we are all responsible for what we decide to do about them. And although I can't quite promise you eternity, I *can* promise you that it doesn't take much to go from a life impaired by bad habits to a life enhanced by good ones.

Because the body loves habits. And it will always be satisfied by the ones you give it. Give it good ones, it will happily adopt them. Give it bad ones, it will bend to them just as compliantly. The body is a bit like a child. If you treat it well, it will reward you a hundredfold, but if you treat it badly you will pay for it later. In matters of health, as in life, in the end you reap what you sow.

I would be embarrassed to trot out such banalities but for the fact that, since taking the Hippocratic Oath more than three decades ago, I have been privileged to observe, on a daily basis, what feeble custodians of our health most of us are.

We tend to think that health is something we are owed, something we have acquired for eternity. That is the Care Bear version of life. In reality, health is capital that should be turned to profit, or at least – let's be realistic – that we should cherish so we don't lose it. Not too quickly anyway . . . Because this capital has a habit of eroding sneakily, one day at a time. If we don't respect it, it silently takes its revenge.

I'm like you. I like loafing on my sofa and giving in to the comfort of doing sod all. I put off until tomorrow the exercise I had planned to do today. Yes, I'm like you: I'm not averse to sugary things and I love a glass of something. Like you, I know that I'd be better off munching on some fruit than putting away a slice of toast and Nutella. Can I swear never to have succumbed to tasty temptations? Of course not. Like you, I understand that a raw vegetable will always be better for me than a handful of peanuts. And yet, like you, with pre-dinner drinks or at a party, with alcohol lending a hand, I reach for a slice of salami here, a pistachio there . . . Because I have got into the habit of associating these things with conviviality and good times. And my body doesn't argue.

One day, a child asked me a question: Why are tasty things bad for you? At the sight of the moronic expression that came over me, he ran a mile, I seem to remember. But the incident forced me to think and to ask some questions of my own: What are we to do? How can we be careful and still enjoy life?

I shook off my moronic expression and decided to come up with a response. That is the purpose of this book. I haven't written it to awaken the paranoid in you, rather to reacquaint you with a few virtuous principles. It takes the form of shortish passages grouped together in four chapters:

– The first chapter is about healthy foods that are sometimes overlooked. I won't just recommend them, I'll tell you why you should eat them and how they are useful to your body. I won't just say: 'Eat clementines!', I'll explain why doing so hugely benefits your physical and mental fitness. And I bet when you next see a clementine on a market stall or in a fruit bowl, you'll think about what you've read and give in to temptation. Safe in the knowledge that you are doing yourself good. And doing ourselves good is always pleasurable, and therefore always rewarding. The same with vegetables. My wish list is subjective, not exhaustive. It could be different. It conveys my preferences, my priorities, my discoveries, and includes nothing but goodness.

– The second chapter focuses on those little habits that either harm or enhance our well-being. Sometimes there is so little separating the two. Not eating rubbish when you're hungover. Not falling into the trap of buying overpriced moisturizers. Or just knowing how to sit properly: it's silly, but if your posture is wrong, you think you're relaxing when in fact you're exerting constant effort that your back won't forget in a hurry. Ah, backache. It wreaks havoc. It should be classified as a road-safety issue. Say two people travel 500km in a car, one sitting badly, one sitting properly. Barring accident, they will both arrive at the same destination, at the same time. But not in the same state. For days, the person whose posture was poor won't feel right. Spasms, backache . . . It could be severe. Or mild. In which case, this person won't pay much attention. So they will do the same again: 500km in the other direction with the same poor posture. In the end, things will deteriorate. And all because, for a few hours, they got into the habit of doing something badly. Doing something well costs nothing, if you can be bothered. You can count on me to tell you how to sit properly at the wheel. And in a chair. And how to stay standing without wrecking your spine. And plenty more besides. Often you will say to yourself: Well, yes, that's *obvious*! In which case, I have sounded the alarm and fulfilled my brief. Just registering good and bad patterns of behaviour, just thinking about them, counts as taking action.

– The third chapter is aimed at the fit person who is snoozing somewhere inside all of us: it will make you want to move more than you do currently. Studies about people's attitudes to exercise are often contradictory but rarely encouraging . . . If I were to recall just one, it would be that of the Eurobarometer (the European Union does like to have its say), which concluded that less than half of the population exercises at least once a week (2014). That is not enough! You don't have to call yourself sporty to do the minimum amount of exercise our bodies require. You will learn that it's possible to be active without even realizing it. I'll point you to forms of exercise you won't have considered, but which are proving more and more popular. I will enliven the conversation about fitness with a host of recommendations that also apply to those of you who exercise regularly. I will quash some common misconceptions (yes, you *do* avoid coffee before a sports session; no, you do *not* buy a pair of trainers without due thought) and I will answer questions I know you ask yourself (about nutrition, effort, recovery), as well as questions you don't ask but will soon realize you should be asking . . .

– The fourth and final chapter groups together several useful bits of advice for keeping in shape. What I call 'the small stuff that does you long-term good', things we need only devote a few minutes to each day, that we can sometimes do while going about our daily business, but that, taken together, will make you feel good and love life. And make it last longer. You will learn how to look after your memory, take care of your heart, prevent constipation, discover that it's okay to sleep at the office and understand once and for all how tobacco and alcohol can take possession of your brain if you let them. Among other things . . .

Our health has a tendency to get knocked off course by draconian diets, restrictive attitudes, endless prescriptions and pharmacies spewing out medicine, when all it needs is a bit of common sense. That's why this book, which has been a long time in the making, is made up of short sections – sometimes very short – that are always accurate and always useful. You might read it in one go but, thereafter, you're bound to dip in and out because it's brimming with practical advice that can be followed straight away. I have deliberately written it in a relaxed style. This shouldn't detract in any way from the seriousness and pertinence of the content. And as I'm convinced that a smile and a laugh are sources of energy and happiness, unlike counterproductive overdramatizing, I couldn't stop myself adding a dash of humour here and there. Sorry, that's the way I am and I shan't change, particularly as my compatriots have been kind enough to tell me, on more than one occasion, that my jokes are just about tolerable.

I prefer to convince people rather than preach to them, charm rather than threaten, inform rather than frighten. I believe there is no right age to start. No right age to take charge. No right age to do yourself good. No right age to take control of your health, or take back control. No right age to say: You know what? This goose isn't cooked!

Healthy foods

The principles of eating well

I'm always saying you have to eat healthily. But what does that actually involve? What are the basic principles to observe if you want to eat well? What will help you get into shape? Here are five simple principles, observe them and you will quickly feel the benefits:

1. **Eat balanced meals** They should contain carbohydrates, of course: you'll find those in grains, preferably wholemeal ones. They should also contain protein: think lentils, beans, chickpeas but also fish and meat, preferably white. Lipids need to be chosen carefully: those found in nuts or olive oil will do you a power of good. Just to remind you, broadly speaking, carbohydrates are sugars and lipids are fats.
2. **Vary your diet** When you eat grains, avoid always going for the same ones. There's more to life than rice and pasta. There are rye crackers, gluten-free flour, cornmeal, quinoa . . . A bit of creativity wouldn't hurt.
3. **Prioritize freshness and good quality** Industrially baked goods and frozen ready-meals are certainly practical, and occasionally tasty too, but they aren't usually very good for your health.

It's not a question of banning them, just consuming them in homeopathic doses . . .

4. **Be sensible** We sometimes get into the habit of having second helpings for no good reason and eating when we aren't hungry. These are the surest ways to stray from a healthy weight. Cut down on portion sizes. And if, for psychological reasons, you feel the need to have a nice full plate in front of you, make cunning adjustments: reduce portions of foods that are high in calories (pasta, rice, etc) and increase portions of foods that are low in calories (vegetables). I even know some people, the really crafty ones, who eat off small plates: they find it satisfying to see a proper plateful when they sit down to eat.

5. **Think flavour** Eating must always be pleasurable. The kings of the food industry have understood as much and snare us with dishes whose salt, sugar and fat contents are all, alas, too high. But it is possible to eat tasty foods without damaging your health. All you have to do is opt for fresh food and go all out on the herbs. There is a plethora of them available and they're stuffed with nutrients to boot.

Garlic, a superfood

Go Gallic, go garlic! It is a welcome addition to hot and cold dishes: meats, salads, soups or pasta. When eaten fresh, whether cooked or raw (raw is best, because its nutritional value is higher), it provides protection against stomach and intestinal cancer. And, although not enough studies on the subject have been carried out yet, we suspect this superfood works wonders for your larynx, your breasts, Madam, and your prostate, Sir (according to research from the Shanghai Cancer Institute).

It really is in your best interests to eat garlic; the list of benefits goes on: it helps battle cardiovascular disease, the effects of ageing (being rich in antioxidants) and is thought to prevent all manner of infections.

Granted, you might read somewhere that Shakespeare did not consider garlic to be a noble food or that Cervantes did not much like the smell. But you'll concede that both these gentlemen had more talent for writing than health matters. With the greatest respect to them both, take my word for it, eating this bulbous plant does you no end of good. As for the famous smell that so inconvenienced Cervantes, there are ways of dealing with it, you know. Not by brushing your teeth after eating (as many people believe) but by chewing on some parsley, fresh mint or coffee beans. Or, even more effective: make your friends eat garlic with you!

Antioxidants act as a sort of shield against free radicals. Each of our cells (the human body is the sum total of billions) breathes. In doing so, it produces oxygen by-products that we term free radicals. Their favourite target? Other human cells. They oxidize them, speeding up the cells' ageing process and, therefore, ours too. The body needs antioxidants to resist this phenomenon. Hence our daily obligation to eat, among other good things, fruit and vegetables, since they contain them in abundance.

The indispensable wheatgerm

Now, vitamin E is a powerful antioxidant. Yes, it protects your cells against the ageing process. Like most people, I imagine you sometimes wonder where it can be found. The answer is simple: in wheatgerm. Not exclusively there, certainly, but very much there . . . Judge for yourself: you only need to swallow two teaspoons of wheatgerm to get a third of your daily dose of vitamin E. It would be a shame not to take advantage, wouldn't you say?

Its capacity to protect us doesn't stop there: in those two fabulous teaspoons you will also find a third of your zinc requirement (helps to protect you from infection as well as to form scabs when the need arises) and a quarter of your magnesium requirement (part of a collection of anti-stress and anti-fatigue minerals). Wait, there's more: wheatgerm is also recommended for combating high cholesterol and promoting good retinal health. I know you'll keep an eye out for it now . . . So all you need to know is how to eat it.

One imperative: do not heat it. This degrades its vitamins and essential fatty acids. Apart from that, go for it! Sprinkle it on your crudités, soups, fruit compotes, yogurts . . . You will find that wheatgerm goes well with sweet and savoury dishes. That's because its taste is neutral. Unlike the influence it will have on your health: that will be entirely positive.

Brewer's yeast: health and beauty in one hit

Spells of fatigue? Irritability? Have you thought of brewer's yeast? You haven't? Give it a try. In capsules or in flakes, powder or tablets, brewer's yeast comes in many different forms and always does your body good. It provides you with proteins, trace elements and vitamins (essentially D and some of the B group) that are guaranteed to detox.

Here's something else to add to the catalogue of benefits: brewer's yeast improves digestion, particularly for pregnant women, who tend to enjoy their very own cocktail of nausea, tummy aches and sometimes vomiting too. Finally, keep in mind that regular consumption is good for your nails, helps hair rediscover its shine and gives skin a healthy glow.

The danger, therefore, is overdosing. As ever, don't overdo it: no more than three teaspoonfuls a day, and take it for short spells rather than all the time. Otherwise? Otherwise, it will have a boomerang effect: your intestinal flora will become imbalanced and you'll be back where you started.

Fonio: 100 per cent grain, 0 per cent gluten

Tired of the same old grains? Prepared to spend a bit more than you do on rice or buckwheat?

Don't delay, try fonio today!

Little known in France, if at all, fonio is probably one of Africa's oldest grains. I'm not going to spin you a line about how great it tastes: it is rather bland. But that aside, the benefits of fonio really stack up. From magnesium to zinc, calcium to manganese, it is packed with micronutrients that are considered good for us. Plus, it is easy to cook, organic (you can only get it in specialist shops) and naturally gluten free. Good news for people who are allergic to gluten or have decided to remove it from their diet (although the gluten-free fad annoys me a bit – see the entry entitled 'Gluten free is doubt-full').

One last thing: fonio is very nourishing but it is also a recommended food for people who are overweight. If that applies to you, try out this grain pronto.

There's no 'arm in an almond!

Right, now we've got that terrible joke out of the way, let us move on to weightier matters. Do, seriously, think of almonds. They contain, along with other nutrients, calcium, proteins and vitamin E, whose antioxidant powers are well known.

But, I hear you say, almonds are high in fat. Yes. But there is fat, and there is fat. Good fat and bad fat. As it happens, almonds are jammed full of good fats called omega-3s and these strapping little fellows know how to keep cholesterol at bay, fight hypertension and do battle with osteoarthritis. All that while beefing up your immune system too.

Another reason why almonds ride high in the charts of dieting excellence is fibre. They are full of it. Benefit number one: they make you feel full. Benefit number two: they aid digestion.

Do not turn into a squirrel. *Do* be aware of the merits of this nut that is handy to carry around, doesn't make a mess and goes extremely well with fruit compotes and vegetable dishes.

Convinced? Go on, it won't even cost you an almond-a-leg . . .

Rooibos: red-tea-tastic

Rooibos . . . If the pronunciation bothers you just say 'redbush': it's the same thing. Why 'red'? Because the leaves tend to turn a purplish-red.

Redbush is drunk as an infusion, hot or cold (or even iced). Its flavour? Fruity and smoky. But it isn't any old herbal tea: it's a drink that helps you sleep better and aids digestion. So much so that in South Africa (where rooibos comes from, inland from Cape Town to be precise) many doctors recommend this tea for relieving colic in babies.

But the charms of this novel drink do not stop there. It contains numerous antioxidants, which, you will recall, are your body's best friend: they protect your organs from some cancers, degenerative diseases, cardiovascular problems and more generally from the effects of ageing.

Of course, new products can become fashionable. In fact, they invariably do. But with rooibos it's justified, since this drink contains neither theine nor caffeine. Consequently, it has fewer side effects. For starters, it doesn't act as a diuretic and get you visiting the smallest room in the house more often than you would like.

Milk is better fermented

In India they call it 'lassi'. In North Africa it is 'leben'. In the Caucasus, 'kefir'. Behind these exotic-sounding names you will find fermented milk. The taste is more acidic and the texture creamier than regular milk. The difference is that lactic acid culture has been added, while preserving milk's nutritional qualities. You'll find it has just as many proteins and carbohydrates and just as much calcium.

The special thing about fermented milk is that it is swarming with living lactic bacteria. Bacteria? That's right, bacteria. Does that alarm you? Well, it needn't (see p. 14). These 'good' bacteria are called probiotics (the term was first used in 1965: make a note and show off to your friends). We recognize them by their resilience and their activity. Resilience because they survive their journey through the gastrointestinal tract. Activity because they are capable of sticking to intestinal cells and multiplying, so as to supplant pathogenic bacteria, the 'bad' ones. They are built to win the bacterial wars that are played out in your body on a daily basis. The result is a better balance of intestinal flora, which can be permanently destabilized by stress, a failing in our diet or even by taking medication.

It is straightforward: fermented milk can be drunk plain or flavoured with a syrup or even with mixed fruits. The important thing is to drink it quickly: these friendly bacteria do not have much patience, and as time passes their numbers decrease. However, you can be clever about it and integrate it into your diet: fermented milk is a good substitute for cream in a sauce or soup (cold, because cooking destroys the bacteria).

As a rule, the mere mention of the word bacteria makes people run a mile. To most people's way of thinking, bacteria = illness. The thing is, some bacteria are your pals. Lifelong friends even. They are **probiotics**. These living micro-organisms help digest lactose (not an easy feat for everyone). Another benefit: they are useful in cases of diarrhoea, for both children and adults, and they will survive a course of antibiotics. Beyond this, the medical fraternity talk in hypotheses. It's possible that probiotics prevent pain and bloating and strengthen the immune system. But these are only suppositions for now. A word of advice: if in doubt, take them. Probiotics can never do you any harm, no matter how many you consume.

The bergamot orange: the forgotten citrus fruit

It's the shape of a pear, looks like an orange, reveals a greenish flesh beneath thick smooth skin, usually yellow, and was introduced into Europe during the Crusades. Either that or Christopher Columbus brought it back from the Canary Islands.

Have you got it yet? Of course you have, the answer's in the heading!

So, the bergamot orange . . . Why tell you about it? Because it's a good idea to discover, or rediscover, a fruit that abounds with health benefits but is sometimes overlooked (so much so that it's hard to come by: try luxury or health-food shops). But first off, I need to say that the bergamot orange is not recommended during the first three months of pregnancy. If this applies to you, turn to the next section and pay this one a visit later.

The bergamot orange acts like a tranquillizer, in the most natural way possible. It boosts the production of melatonin, the hormone that regulates our body clock, so it can be a great help in cases of insomnia or jet lag.

In addition, the bergamot is a trusty friend to your stomach. It stimulates digestion and relieves stomach cramps, even those caused by stress or anxiety.

Finally, it might be handy to know that bergamot oranges can be used to combat psoriasis (a non-contagious skin disorder characterized by red lesions) and prevent hyperactivity.

So, plenty of reasons to find some room for the bergamot orange in your life. After all, it can be consumed in hundreds of ways: reach for one in a fruit bowl or have a cup of tea flavoured with it; and you will also find it in various skin creams or bottles of essential oils.

Baobab

If you haven't already heard of baobab – sometimes called 'monkey bread' – then you will soon. It is one of many novel foods turning up in our culinary culture with the official stamp of 'healthy'.

Behind this rather odd-sounding name you will actually find . . . a fruit. Of the baobab tree. You can eat it in ready-made powder form or crush the dried pulp from the fruit (if you can find it). Either way, you can sprinkle it on cereal or yogurt, add it to a smoothie, or use it in baking or sauces. And that's just for starters . . .

Of course, the aim of the game is not to eat baobab fruit just so you can boast about eating baobab fruit, though it is extremely trendy. Monkey bread owes its success, in part, to its high vitamin C content: six times greater than that of the orange. It also contains twice as much calcium as milk, as well as phosphorus, iron and, to cap it all, enough antioxidants to be recommended eating for anyone who is worried about getting old: a legitimate concern, if you ask me! Lastly, this 'new' food helps you concentrate and recover after exercise.

Lemon: detox ace

Its sourness stimulates the taste buds and aids digestion. Along with other citrus fruits, it is thought to prevent certain cancers (oesophagus, stomach, colon, mouth, larynx, etc), reduce the risk of heart disease and possess anti-inflammatory properties.

At 19 calories per 100g, the lemon is a veritable detox ace. You can have it first thing in the morning, on an empty stomach.

Straight! Or watered down for the more sensitive palate. True, it does give you quite a kick, but it's a great way to get the liver secreting bile so that it's prepared for quality digestion throughout the day.

A freshly squeezed juice will work wonders for your figure and blow away the cobwebs, since lemon is rich in vitamin C. A few mouthfuls, that's all you need to stimulate your renal activity. Lemon's diuretic qualities help expel retained water. In other words, this often neglected fruit is one of your best allies in the fight against cellulite.

Once you start, you're caught in a virtuous cycle. Lemon is a natural hunger suppressant that stabilizes blood sugar levels. When you drink it, you send out a message of fullness that reduces your appetite. If your appetite alarms you, try drinking lemon juice before meals. See for yourself: it calms things down.

Pomegranate – the explosive fruit

Did you know that the term 'hand grenade' comes from the French for pomegranate? You do now.

A glowing assessment of *la grenade* could start with a load of clever words such as 'anthocyanins' and 'ellagic acid', just two of the numerous antioxidants this magic fruit contains. Yes, magic: not content with being nourishing, it is curative too. The tastiest medicine there is.

For starters, the pomegranate is able to clear your coronary arteries of all the fatty deposits that are found there. All right, maybe 'all' is a slight exaggeration. That would make it the best available treatment for heart attacks, which it obviously isn't. Let's just say, it does a spot of housework in your arteries. It helps protect you from atherosclerosis, the excess of bad cholesterol that, along with stress, can lead to hypertension. Pomegranate helps promote elasticity in your arteries and this improves the heart's blood flow. Ultimately, it reduces your risk of having a heart attack.

But that's not all. Stuffed full of vitamins (notably C), the pomegranate boasts a lengthy list of attributes, including the ability to fight cataract growth, strengthen bone and muscles, eliminate intestinal parasites and even reduce dental plaque. To sum up: in juice form or as it comes, this is the fruit of champions. And I'm not employing a sporting term for the hell of it: the pomegranate is an excellent recovery food for fitness fans, since it works against the free radicals and acidity they produce during exercise.

As for the clever clogs who think they can give pomegranate a miss and replace it with a few grenadine cordials – as in *la grenade*, right? – I'll stop you there. There are a few artisan drink-makers who use pulped pomegranates to make grenadine, but you have to get up pretty early in the morning to find one. Most cordials on the market contain some red fruits (redcurrant, raspberry) and a lot of artificial flavouring, colouring and citric acid. So remember: pomegranate is an explosive fruit, grenadine is a damp squib.

Eat clementines!

China is the world's biggest producer. French ones usually come from Corsica. And it is the fourth most eaten fruit in France. It is, of course, the clementine, the ultimate winter fruit: good for morale and a good antidote to bouts of fatigue. It has many attributes, including:

1. **Vitamin C** Swallow just two clementines to get 40mg worth, half the recommended daily dose in the UK, and all you need to feel invigorated, fight fatigue and protect yourself from germs.
2. **Calorie content** It's low. Less than 50 calories per 100g of this sweet, juicy, thirst-quenching citrus fruit.
3. **Mineral salts and trace elements** Its calcium content will delight your bone cells, its magnesium and iron contents strengthen your muscular and nervous systems.
4. **Fibre** Their nutritional value rivals their sweetness. Clementines give your digestion a boost.

As you can see, the list of advantages is long. Clementines are slightly impractical, as it is best to keep them in your fridge's vegetable tray (to stop them drying out). You can reuse the skin, provided you buy untreated fruit. Grated peel makes a delightful addition to home-made cakes.

One last thing, the clementine also gives you an opportunity to lord it over your friends. As you peel one under their envious gaze, explain that the clementine was created in Oran, Algeria, by a missionary called Brother Clément. Hence its name.

Plums matter

Black, red, mauve or yellow, they come in a choice of colours. A raw plum is a fruit with high antioxidant qualities (so it's excellent for doing battle with potentially cancerous cells). And it contains a profusion of vitamins (A, K and particularly C), all of which have their uses. Vitamin A is integral to vision (notably night vision), contributes to healthy skin and mucous membranes and also regulates your immune system, which will be all the more stimulated for the top-up of vitamin C you've just given it. As for vitamin K, that helps fight osteoporosis and facilitates blood clotting.

To enjoy the full flavour of raw plums, they must be just ripe enough. How can you tell? *Simplissime*: check they are soft at either end. They aren't? Wait a while longer, leaving the plums at room temperature. They are? Eat them right away or put them in the fridge, where they will wait patiently for you. You need to get them out a few hours before eating to give the fruit time to recover its maximum flavour.

Lastly, be aware that raw plums, being rich in fibre, have laxative properties. I am duty-bound to inform you . . .

Grapefruit's forbidden past

Have you ever tasted of the Forbidden Fruit? Chances are you have, in more ways than one. An eighteenth-century visitor to Barbados came across a hybrid citrus – a cross between the sweet orange and the pomelo – and thought it was so delicious he decided to name it after the fruit that spelled disaster for Adam and Eve.

But grapefruit certainly shouldn't be forbidden to you. Not least because it is a practical fruit that keeps for a week at room temperature and up to six weeks in the fridge (provided you place it in a closed container).

And that's not all: grapefruit is refreshing, a sure-fire winner when the sun is beating down. Next, it's bursting with vitamin C and we all know how indispensable that is. Lastly, it contains antioxidant compounds that all research suggests are good for you, notably for preventing certain types of cancer. One last thing: grapefruit is highly recommended for people who are overweight.

Grapefruit has so many good qualities that people sometimes forget to specify that it is incompatible with some medication. Lots of people are unaware of this. If you are undergoing treatment (as happens from time to time) mention that you eat grapefruit to your doctor or pharmacist; they will be able to tell you if this fruit, remarkable in every other way, could cause unwelcome effects. It might be temporarily forbidden after all.

Melon, all good

The melon: here is a fruit that has every right to have a big head, seeing how many plus points it has. Whether orange, green or yellow, melons are refreshing, rehydrating and contain a heap of mineral salts that are essential for bones and the proper functioning of your heart, nerves and muscles. Consider too that a single 100g slice provides 10 per cent of your recommended daily dose of vitamin C, and you can see what a positive impact melon has on your immune system (we all know one slice is rarely enough . . .).

There are a thousand reasons for eating melon. Among them, the fact that it protects and softens blood vessels and improves circulation: the kind of thing that prevents heart disease. Melon is also very good for kidney and intestinal function. I will spare you the medical intricacies, but being potassium-rich and sodium-poor gives it diuretic properties. Put simply, it cleans the body by boosting the elimination of waste products. Finally, and less widely known, melon protects your eyes. It contains plenty of beta-carotene so enhances irrigation, reduces the risk of dry eyes and helps you see better during the day and night.

In fact, the only problem with melon is knowing what to serve it with. It's good on its own. But with cured ham to provide some protein, something like prosciutto (preferably with the fat removed), it's even better. Try it in a soup with lemongrass: the combination is said to ease digestive problems. Or, mix it with cucumber in juice form: your kidneys will love you.

Watermelon: eat irresponsibly

The great thing about watermelon, jokers will tell you, is that you wash your hands while you eat. This juiciest of fruits is not only thirst quenching, it is also stuffed full of lycopene, an antioxidant belonging to the carotenoid family (this clever-sounding term refers to the orange pigment that gives carrots their colour). A flurry of benefits ensues: clever old watermelon is thought to reduce our risk of cancer, fight cholesterol and prevent inflammation. Even those little black pips deserve to be swallowed: they contain vitamin C.

Just the small matter of 'watermelon ethics' to discuss. You need a sense of timing and a knack for choosing the right accompaniment. First, from the moment you plunge a knife into your watermelon, you have four days to finish it. Otherwise, the lycopene content drops. And it would be a shame to miss out on all those antioxidants. Secondly, it has been proved that watermelon's goodness is more easily absorbed by the body when you eat it with lipids. Also (and this little secret shall bind us together always) it's in your interest to serve watermelon with a few nuts and a piece of cheese. On paper not an easy task, I grant you, but highly recommended from a biological point of view.

The fruit, the whole fruit and nothing but the fruit

Fruit or fruit juice? We sometimes think the two are of equal value and we are wrong. The body metabolizes them differently.

What is juice? Sugar, water and vitamins. The drink is divested of a large part of the fibre that is present in the fruit when we bite into it. Fancy an apple? Let's take one as an example . . .

Munch on an unpeeled apple (having given it a rinse) and you'll ingest a whole stack of antioxidant compounds because the skin contains more of these than the flesh. These compounds are known to be useful for fighting the effects of ageing and protecting our hearts. They also help build up our defences against cancer. The same applies to fibre, which aids digestion and protects our blood vessels: it is abundant in the skin.

Fibre's distinctive feature? It slows down the arrival of the fruit's sugar (and there is plenty of it) into the blood. That's why our blood glucose levels rocket when we drink a fruit juice. The *British Medical Journal* has even gone as far as suggesting that if we eat the whole fruit we are protecting ourselves from diabetes, whereas we expose ourselves to it by only opting for the juice.

To sum up, it is not forbidden to enjoy a fruit juice from time to time. Freshly squeezed. But don't think of it as a substitute for eating fruit, which has different nutritional qualities and obliges you to chew, a great aid to digestion in itself.

The raisin: an ugly friend

Small, shrivelled, shapeless, withered . . . Objectively, like their sultana cousins, raisins aren't great lookers. But they taste good! And they are good for you. You cannot imagine the number of properties that are crammed into a raisin . . .

For starters, they have formidable antioxidant powers, which will slow down your cells' ageing process. I won't list all the phenols here, but they are jam-packed with resveratrol, the scientific name for a compound that is thought to protect your heart, assuming you have a healthy lifestyle in the first place.

Secondly, in a raisin you will find four times more trace elements than in grapes. Calcium, iron, magnesium, potassium, mineral salts, carbohydrates (I'll come back to them) and a decent amount of vitamin B. All this cannot fail to strengthen your body.

Thirdly, you have to say, the raisin is the ultimate practical fruit. Available throughout the year, easy to store, easy to carry around and easy to gobble on the hoof. But you can also eat them cooked: for a first course, they enhance a salad; for a main course, they go well with fish, meat and poultry; for dessert, they can embellish cookies and pastries. And so on: these fellows have a knack of turning up everywhere, accompanying pre-dinner drinks or in a loaf of bread.

To recap, if you haven't already, take a punt on the raisin. Some people will object, saying they have a high sugar content. Too high, even . . . It is widely accepted that sugar from fruit is not fattening – or only very slightly – and raisins provide welcome energy for mental and physical activity.

Kale and hearty

Kale is in vogue. In the United States they are crazy for it and, as we know, when the Americans adopt something it isn't long before it shows up here. When a few transatlantic stars promoted this curly brassica it was instantly back in fashion. Yes, back: kale was eaten in some European countries in the Middle Ages.

This vegetable, which fell out of favour after the Second World War, is related to broccoli and is, it must be said, packed with good properties: good on a nutritional level, good for your figure and good for your health.

In every 100g of kale, there is close to 120mg of vitamin C (three times more than an orange). I shan't overwhelm you with figures, but it's worth knowing that all manner of goodness is crammed into kale: it contains vitamins A and B6, potassium and calcium (so it's ideal for children, who tend to overdose on dairy products).

Kale is also your figure's best friend. Not content with being ridiculously low in calories, it is also high in fibre. Incredibly high. So much so, that it acts as a hunger suppressant and will keep you away from the fridge.

Lastly, I know I have been banging on about vegetables being good at preventing cancer but kale really is top dog in this regard: good for the prostate, good for the bladder, good for the colon. And, as if that wasn't enough, kale is a powerful antioxidant too: it helps fight cholesterol and heart disease.

The virtuous humble radish

Care about your cardiovascular health? I care about mine. Keen to protect yourself from cancer? Me too. To maximize our chances, we should eat cruciferous vegetables as regularly as possible. And what are they? Turnips, kohlrabi, cauliflowers, broccoli and radishes. Let's dwell on this last one.

The red or white radish is crunchy and refreshing and has a subtle hot flavour. We shouldn't neglect it, not when it has such brilliant antioxidant properties. What's good about the radish is that the whole thing is edible: even the leaves. And you can eat it raw or cooked.

Raw, radishes are a great pre-dinner nibble or addition to a salad. You won't find better accompaniments for tuna, avocado, tomato, boiled eggs or corn on the cob. Plenty of choice there. And they can also be grated or mixed with unsalted butter as a topping for a tart.

You can cook red radishes whole. They only need to be steamed for quarter of an hour, or try frying them in a butter and orange-juice sauce. Simple, tasty and just one of many serving suggestions at your disposal.

With the **radish** nothing is wasted, you can eat the lot. The tops can be cooked like spinach or combined with onion, potatoes, chicken stock and a bit of cream to make a soup. And if sweating over a hot stove bores you rigid, you can just sprinkle them finely chopped over soups and omelettes.

Fennel: eat it with your eyes closed

Obviously, fennel isn't very sexy. I mean, it rhymes with 'kennel' for starters, and such things can put people off . . . However, if you look beyond such phonetic considerations, you stand to gain. Because do you know what? Fennel is very good for you.

Yes, it's good for bone health, good at combating hypertension and good at preventing certain types of cancer, notably colon cancer. Or at least that is what we've gleaned from various experiments carried out on animals that were more or less consenting, frankly. And we reckon what is good for them shouldn't do us lowly humans any harm: we are mammals first and foremost – mammals who understand that if there is the merest whiff of a health benefit we would be foolish to miss out.

Try it, if you're unsure: you'll see that fennel's aniseed flavour is a taste sensation when served with fish or shellfish. There is nothing stopping you putting it in a salad too. And fennel goes splendidly with boiled spuds and red pepper topped off with sweet onion and lemon zest. Fancy adding some prosciutto? Why not . . . But don't go overboard.

While serving **fennel**, don't forget to mention casually to your fellow diners that the word 'fennel' comes from the Old English *finul*, first recorded in the eleventh century and that, in turn, comes from the Latin *faeniculum* meaning 'small hay'. In those days, it was used for repelling insects.

Vegetables: raw or cooked?

Your goose isn't cooked: we established that in the introduction. But what about your carrots? And all your other veg for that matter?

There is no blanket rule. Cooking carrots is a good idea because the cooking process breaks down their cellular lining, facilitating the body's absorption of the carotenoid antioxidants they contain. It's the same with tomatoes: putting them in the oven enhances them nutritionally. When you cook a tomato, you raise its lycopene levels, a useful antioxidant that reduces the risk of cancer and heart problems.

Carrots and tomatoes then, but also broccoli, cabbages, turnips, radishes and most leafy vegetables . . . There are plenty of examples of vegetables that are healthier when cooked.

However, because life isn't simple, it's no good being a cook-it zealot. Raw also has its advantages: to start with, it preserves the numerous vitamins and enzymes that won't survive a dip in the saucepan. And eating raw demands chewing. More chewing for longer. Chewing is good for you! And very good for your stomach: it means some of its work is done in advance. This avoids it overworking, which is usually responsible for the post-meal slump you feel. Bear in mind that the more you chew, the more histamine is secreted by the body. That's the hormone that makes you feel full and stops you stuffing yourself beyond all reason.

To recap, do not abandon cooked in favour of raw or vice versa. Vary the way you serve vegetables, and remember that the most important thing is to eat them regularly.

Fruit 'n' Veg 'n' Kids

Ah, the children! How can you get fruit and vegetables into them? When you say: 'This is healthy, it will make you grow, it will make you big and strong, it's full of vitamins,' they just give you a mocking sneer: 'Oh yeah? Fascinating . . .'

Faced with such obstruction, you have to use cunning ruses:

1. **Give them the illusion of choice** Tomatoes or cucumber? Peas or green beans? Apricots or melon? And so on. Usually the child in question will pull a face then choose what they consider the 'least worst' option. But at least their words are acted upon. You can serve up 'their choice', smiling broadly.

2. **Get them drinking** Present them with fruit and veg in the form of home-made juices, smoothies or cold soups. If a little effort is put into the presentation (i.e. it's served in a fancy glass with a straw), this can really work.

3. **Play with the scale** A child is small. And portions can be presented as miniature versions of the fruit and vegetables themselves. Get the idea? I have never really understood why, but sticks of cucumber or carrot for dipping in fromage frais are more appealing to children than round slices in a dressing.

4. **Stick a chef's hat on their head** What happens if you suggest they help you cook? It doesn't always work, but sometimes this approach draws them in. They'll be keen to eat what they've made and won't want to feel all their work was for nothing.

Saffron: in a golden mood

Have you known happier times? Are your spirits low? I won't claim I can fix the problem with a few sentences in a book, but I will give you pathways to follow that, over time, can help you battle depression. One of these paths is via food and specifically a spice that is not only tasty but has a well-earned reputation for lifting one's spirits too: saffron.

This spice is found in numerous cultures and civilizations, going back five thousand years. It is sometimes used for medicinal purposes too. Saffron's energizing qualities give the spirits a lift. And not just the spirits! Some people insist that a modest but regular consumption of saffron won't do your libido any harm either . . .

My advice: use it in thread rather than powder form. It will enhance a paella, stew, risotto or bouillabaisse marvellously.

Now you're convinced, there is just one rather irksome matter to discuss: the price. Do you know the other name for saffron? Red gold . . . In other words, it ain't cheap. Not cheap at all: around €3000 for 100g. I can hear you spluttering. But you don't need tons of it. One gram can be used for dozens of meals.

Saffron is worth a lot of money because it is difficult to extract. The meticulous process is done by hand and is, therefore, time-consuming. That doesn't deter people from getting into the saffron business, mind you. More and more are doing so, which shows that demand is rising. Thirty years ago, there were only a few saffron makers in France. Today, you can find hundreds, most of them based in the Provence-Alpes-Côte d'Azur region.

The forgotten virtues of cinnamon

Unless I'm very much mistaken, you don't like germs. That is something we have in common . . . To take the fight to them on a daily basis, and give yourself a treat, you have a friend at your disposal: cinnamon. In ancient Egypt, well before our time, it was used to embalm the dead. Later, the European nobility used it to mask the unpleasant taste of some foods. Today, as an infusion, it is credited with having miraculous powers thanks to its exceptional antibacterial qualities.

A preface: cinnamon is not recommended for pregnant women or people with cardiac arrhythmia or gastritis. For everyone else, this is a five-star spice. The Ministry of Health should hand it out for free; I am *this* close to starting a petition actually.

Cinnamon protects your digestive system. It will make you less prone to 'stomach heaviness' or diarrhoea. And, taken as an infusion or added to food, it helps regulate blood sugar levels. Thanks to its high antioxidant levels, cinnamon also helps you fight heart disease, which, contrary to popular belief, concerns women as much as men. Finally, note this handy double whammy: it combats genital infections *and* reduced libido (some people even call it an aphrodisiac). Neat, eh?

Put a bit of heart into your diet

Taking care of your heart is a sure-fire way to set in motion a cascade of benefits for the rest of the body. A healthy heart is good for the brain, good for the kidneys, good for muscles, good for everything! All our organs depend on the heart for oxygenation and nutrition. Specifically, a healthy heart leads to:

- feeling younger physically
- an end to shortness of breath after the slightest physical effort
- a longer life with a better quality

What does your little heart need? Love, obviously. But that's not all . . . To continue beating steadily, this most precious of organs also requires healthy food. And cuisine-wise you have to be on your guard because it knows how to distinguish between friend and foe.

On the friendly side, I implore you to eat fish. There is nothing remotely fishy about fish (thanks for squeezing out a smile). It contains healthy fats and comes in a wide variety of flavours, from salmon to herring, from mackerel to sardines via halibut. Of course, you should always favour poaching it in a seasoned stock or baking it in a foil parcel, over frying.

Some meats are heart-friendly: poultry is rich in unsaturated fats, which are better for your heart than their saturated cousins; eating poultry instead of fattier meat may help to reduce your levels of bad cholesterol.

Vegetables provide unadulterated goodness, I can't say it enough, and as for oils, take your pick from the vegetable varieties: soybean, olive, rapeseed or sunflower. They are all useful for your arteries.

Having looked over the 'friends', it is time to assess the 'foes'. It would take hours to draw up an exhaustive list . . . These are the most salient main culprits: cold meats, pastries, butter, cream and cheese (particularly hard ones) do not have entirely good intentions. Meat-wise, be careful with mutton, lamb and beef, which are bursting with saturated fats, the ones we should avoid. And I'm not all that keen on people eating processed meat such as bacon and sausages.

To quote a sixties French slogan: 'Forbidding is forbidden.'

Don't ban any foods but, as always, don't overdo it when faced with excess. And that includes an excess of inactivity. A good diet will give you energy and get-up-and-go. The opposite is true of a high-fat diet, which is detrimental to the heart and will keep you glued to your sofa.

What are the **heavy metals** people often mention in relation to sea and freshwater fish? They exist, but don't panic... Since the beginning of the industrial age, humans have been discarding mercury into rivers and oceans. Who lives in these waters? Fish. Who eats in these waters? Fish. Who swallows the mercury? Fish. And who eats the fish? You. Me. Us. At least, we are strongly advised to. We know that mercury is toxic for the brain, and that is why the French Agency for Food Safety recommends we limit ourselves to two portions of fish a week. That leaves you with a choice: monkfish, bass, bream, tuna, halibut . . . Salmon is also affected, not because of its mercury content but rather its level of dioxins, substances that are found in freshwater fish. But the guidelines leave plenty of wriggle room . . . By eating these foods regularly, but not obsessively, you only risk one thing: having a nice full tank of omega-3s and vitamins.

Omega-3s? Yes, but . . .

For years now, influenced by magazines and a desire to keep up with the latest trends, people have been queuing up to extol the virtues of omega-3s. And that is no bad thing: as well as being anti-inflammatory and blood thinning, omega-3s regulate cell growth. They are extremely good for you. I can confirm it is important to prioritize foods that are rich in them: oily fish, rape-seed oil, nuts, meat, milk and eggs, the most organically produced you can find. However, a classic error is to stuff yourself with omega-3s, with a nice clean conscience, without taking steps to look after other aspects of your diet.

The thing is, omega-3 has an evil twin brother: omega-6. They both belong to the family of polyunsaturated fatty acids. They are both crucial for the body, although omega-6 is pro-inflammatory and pro-coagulant. Here's where things get tricky: to be metabolized by the body, omega-3s and omega-6s require a common enzyme. And if there is an excess of omega-6s, they monopolize this enzyme. Meaning the omega-3s aren't used by the body, which is, I'm sure you will agree, unfortunate. To recap, eating omega-3s is good, but you have to think about simultaneously reducing your consumption of omega-6s. To do this, you can limit your use of corn and sun-flower oil, both of which are far too prevalent in westerners' diets.

Farmed fish or wild fish? Rather than choosing one over the other, you're best off embracing both. Which doesn't mean they have the same nutritional qualities. The well-fed farmed fish contains fat: good fat (omega-3) and less good fat (omega-6) if the fat content of its diet is too high, which can happen. But it is still rich in vitamins. A wild fish wakes up in the morning without knowing what it is going to eat. It hoovers up what it finds, so it can't guarantee to offer a wealth of omega-3s. But its flesh is firmer and it has more taste than its farmed colleague. So, which is it to be? Alternate . . .

Peanut butter: a good substitute

Do you like the taste of peanut butter? Hardly surprising. But it frightens you? That's not surprising either. Butter is wicked, right? And peanuts are devilishly bad for you, aren't they? So peanut butter must be positively satanic, the alliance of two scourges, the merging of two mortal sins. However . . .

I'll keep it short: yes, peanut butter contains fat. But crossing it off your shopping list could be a mistake. Careful now, I am not encouraging you to stuff yourself with it, just asking you to consider using it instead of other fatty substances. Because peanut butter can replace butter (when making a sauce or even a cake) and be a substitute for oil (in a salad dressing or a wok). The figures speak for themselves: 100g of peanut butter contain 640 calories, versus 730 for butter and 900 for oil.

If you are tempted to give it a try, bear in mind that you are better off heading for the organic range. Here you will find products that contain less sugar and salt and often no palm oil. But once again, the idea is to use peanut butter as a replacement for, not a supplement to, even fattier products.

What if you crack? Feel the urge to treat yourself to a little supplement after all? In that case, spread it (thinly) on a slice of wholemeal bread, which will have the advantage of boosting your fibre and mineral intake.

I eat and I have a flat stomach

Ah, those little bulges inherited from winter, or even spring. When summer blooms, we dream of having a flat stomach. We never think of ourselves as 'just right' in this department.

What happens if, instead of forbidding yourself things, for once you give yourself permission? You give yourself permission to eat, just not to eat any old rubbish? Mother Nature offers plenty of resources that can be allies to your slender self. Some foods are so low in calories that you can eat them to your heart's content. They are nutritional and will reduce your appetite for that dangerous moment when pudding is served.

Among them, unsurprisingly, we find all the leafy vegetables: chard, cabbage and so on. Keep telling yourself one thing: if it's green, chances are it's good for you. I strongly advise you to eat them at home (simmered in stock) rather than in a restaurant, where they quite often arrive drowned in butter.

Without detailing the virtues of each and every one, we can list the foods that deserve a place in your larder when the swimsuit time of year comes around (and even a bit before, because you're better off thinking ahead . . .).

Here they are: turkey breast, brown rice, oat flakes, ginger, cucumber, artichoke, asparagus, avocado (not too many, it is calorific), almonds (not too many, for the same reason). Drinks-wise: green tea, freshly squeezed lemon juice, peppermint tea (a really invigorating flavour). And melon, mango and pineapple . . . And raspberries, whole or crushed, which are an excellent replacement for sugar in your fromage frais (low fat, if you please). This list is not exhaustive. But you'll agree, there is already plenty to enjoy while sparing the bulge. And if, on top of that goodness, you treat yourself to a few sessions on your abdominals, you will quickly see the results . . .

A look at the paleo diet

Unless you live in a cave, you will have heard of the paleo diet. It is an eye-catching and original idea that is attracting more and more followers.

This diet involves eating like prehistoric man. At least as regards the contents of your plate. Tools-wise, you can keep your knife and fork. And you can still wash your hands before a meal too.

Cavemen were gatherers first and foremost. So, the paleo diet suggests eating seasonal (organic) vegetables and fruit.

Cavemen were thieves: they stole from birds' nests. So, the paleo diet includes eggs.

Cavemen were hunters. But sometimes they came back empty-handed. So, lean meat is okay (chicken, game, veal, etc), alternated with fish (because cavemen were also fishermen).

Cavemen were foodies. Enough so, at least, for the experts to allow you seeds and nuts, which have antioxidant properties and provide vegetable and mineral protein. So get eating pumpkin and sunflower seeds, macadamia nuts, pistachios, pine nuts and so on. In reasonable quantities, as ever.

Cavemen were a bit bear-like: they loved honey. On the paleo diet, do the same; use honey to sweeten your desserts.

You will appreciate that there were no cereal crops in the Paleolithic Era, no dairy products, no potatoes and no mass-produced goods: so all these are off limits if you're doing the paleo diet.

About the Mediterranean diet

It is also called the Cretan diet, for the simple reason that people who live in Crete have the world's lowest cardiovascular mortality rate. This diet claims to be your heart's best friend. The European Society of Cardiology agrees: it recommends the Mediterranean diet and says it forms an integral part of any heart treatment. Alongside regular exercise, it helps to keep the cardiovascular system healthy. It also prevents heart attacks and strokes.

The Mediterranean diet has the twin advantage of being varied and easy to observe. Its rules are straightforward:

- Meat does not figure very much: animal protein is chiefly provided by poultry, eggs, fish and dairy products, particularly from goats and sheep, and these should be consumed in moderation, i.e. each item two or three times a week.
- Fish is given priority (being rich in heart-protecting omega-3s). You have to eat it at least once a week, ideally two or even three times, and oily fish (tuna, salmon, sardines, mackerel, etc) are preferred, whether fresh (always better) or tinned.
- Fruit and vegetables should be eaten in large quantities (daily) for their antioxidant properties. In terms of vegetables, leeks, tomatoes, courgettes, aubergines, salads and the cabbage family (Savoy cabbage, broccoli, Brussels sprouts) receive a hearty welcome . . .
- Garlic, onions, spices and seasonings feature virtually all the time. A dish that does not include them would be highly suspect!
- Olive oil is inescapable: it is the go-to fat.
- Sugary foods? No reason why not, but in moderation: no question of having them every day.
- Add a daily intake of nuts or seeds, wholemeal grains, then wash it all down with a glass of red wine, and you are adhering to the main principles of a supposedly miraculous diet. You did read that right: a glass of red wine . . . Not a glass after every mouthful. Otherwise, your heart might be all right but you'll have trouble with your other organs, the liver for one.

Bear in mind that the **Mediterranean diet** comes as a whole: ignoring some of its rules will reduce its effectiveness. Also, as the name suggests, it has evolved for populations who live near the Mediterranean and benefit from sunshine that guarantees them vitamin D provision, which is reduced in murkier climes. Consequently, those who are a little less spoilt weather-wise need to get their vitamin D from additional oily fish (salmon, sardines, mackerel) or make do with dairy products fortified with vitamin D.

Ten suggestions for fat burning

Do you think you're carrying a bit of fat? Get it working. Mobilize it by eating the right things. It will go away of its own accord.

Okay, that's a rather sweeping statement, but there is something in it: some foods do burn fat. They have the triple benefits of facilitating digestion, making you feel full and stimulating the metabolism. By prioritizing them (the foods, not the fats), you will slow down the fat-storing mechanism and prevent it going into overdrive. Here are ten such foods:

1. **Zero-fat and high-protein dairy products** Have them for breakfast and your body will require energy to digest them: it draws on existing reserves and burns calories. These products will stop you feeling peckish at 11am, too.
2. **Oat bran** It is well established that oat bran makes you feel full, because it's rich in fibre. The fibre also slows down the absorption of sugar into the blood, which helps avoid the

peaks and troughs in energy that get us ferreting around in the cupboard or fridge towards the end of the morning. Plus, oat bran goes perfectly with dairy products, whose praises I sang just a few lines above. Ideal for breakfast.

3. **Chilli** The minute you eat some chilli, your body's internal temperature rises. The metabolism is given a boost. Mind you, it doesn't half burn . . . So, don't be too heavy-handed.

4. **Cinnamon** Adding cinnamon to your food is a way of reducing and stabilizing blood sugar levels. Sugar makes you put on weight. So, less sugar = less weight (a neat equation, I think you'll agree).

5. **Vinegar** This also helps regulate blood sugar levels. Don't try it by the glass, it's better on a salad . . .

6. **Lean meat, fish, eggs and so on** As long as you continue eating protein (strongly recommended), it will continue requiring energy to be digested. This is precisely what the foods listed above provide. Over to you.

7. **Lemons** They contain citric acid, which helps burn fat. A small glass of juice first thing in the morning will do you the world of good.

8. **Apples** Eaten as a snack, they cleverly trap some lipids before they turn into fat rolls.

9. **Green tea** People are forever praising its slimming and diuretic effect. Tannins reduce fat absorption.

10. **Coffee** For coffee read caffeine. It has benefits, namely it burns some fats. Watch out for the boomerang effect though: no more than three cups a day or you risk succumbing to anxiety or stress that often result in . . . guess what? Fat storing!

Because you can buy them without prescription, **food sup-plements** are not considered medication. Does that mean they are harmless? No. Can they cause undesirable side effects? Yes. Which is why, if you feel the need to take them, you should consult your doctor first. Alternatively, of course, you could opt simply to adjust your diet instead, which would be more sensible. If you believe you are short of zinc, magnesium, iron, vitamin C or whatever, may I remind you they are all contained in everyday foods. Which are healthy and freely available. You just have to resolve to go and get them . . .

Vitamins: where and why?

Vitamin is a magic word! I'm always telling viewers of my television show not to go short of vitamins. I've probably started to bore people with endless talk of vitamins A, B, C, D, etc. It's not surprising it all gets a bit confusing. What are they for? Where can you find them?

Don't panic! I suggest we review them all:

1. **Vitamin A** is good for vision, bone growth and healthy skin. And it protects us from infection. We find it in offal, herring and a whole raft of vegetables, including sweet potato, carrot, spinach, cabbage and squashes.
2. **Vitamin C** is very good for bone health, cartilage, teeth and gums, it protects us from infection and speeds up scab formation. Its antioxidant properties are established beyond all doubt. It can be found in numerous vegetables (broccoli, red

pepper, beetroot) and a great many fruits (orange, strawberry, kiwi, mango, guava, blackcurrants).

3. **Vitamin D** is essential for healthy bones and teeth. It also plays a role in cell growth, particularly cells associated with the immune system. A shortage can lead to heart disease and cancers. We synthesize this vitamin by exposing ourselves to sunlight: UV rays transform certain skin molecules into vitamin D. But we don't get enough sunshine during the summer to stock up for the rest of the year. That is why many of us are deficient in vitamin D. You can get it from beef liver, cows' milk and fish (salmon, red tuna, pickled herring and sardines).

4. **Vitamin E** is good for the heart and has anti-inflammatory properties. It can be found in almonds, hazelnuts, wholemeal grains and avocados.

5. **Vitamin K** plays an important role in blood clotting. It can be found in green vegetables (spinach, broccoli, Brussels sprouts, asparagus, lettuce, green beans, peas) and also in kiwis.

Vitamin B: a big family

The more attentive among you will have noticed the absence of vitamin B from the previous entry. But it is every bit as important as the others. Though I should say 'they are', not 'it is', since the vitamin Bs constitute a large family. There is a plethora of them: it all depends what number they go by. Let's review these too:

1. **Vitamin B1** is involved with growth and energy production. Plus, it helps with the transmission of nerve impulses. It can be found in pork, wheatgerm, wholemeal grains and certain fruit and vegetables, such as oranges and peas.

2. **Vitamin B2** plays a role in energy production, like its pal vitamin B1. But we also need it for making red blood cells and hormones and for some tissue repair. It can be found in poultry, molluscs, eggs, dairy products and walnuts.

3. **Vitamin B3** facilitates normal health and development. Like the previous two, it plays a part in energy production. Find it in liver, roast chicken, veal escalope, tuna, salmon, cod and wholemeal grain products.

4. **Vitamin B5** helps fight stress, among its other roles. At home in varied and multiple foods: meat, salmon, cod, hard-boiled eggs, offal, mushrooms, sunflower seeds, etc.

5. **Vitamin B6** Going without would disrupt your mental balance. But it has other functions too: it helps make red blood cells and regulates blood sugar levels. Want some? Find it in poultry, fish, tinned chickpeas, liver and sesame and sunflower seeds.

6. **Vitamin B8** If I tell you it is needed for transforming compounds such as glucose and fats, you might zone out. Just trust me: it's important. You would do well to eat fish, cauliflower, liver, offal, egg yolks and soya.

7. **Vitamin B9** is also called the pregnancy vitamin. So, this one is for you if you're waiting for a certain exciting event to occur. It has thousands of functions: it protects against certain congenital defects, is involved with human cell production and plays a role in making DNA and in the working of the nervous and immune systems. Plus, your body's tissue repair on the day of the birth will be thanks to B9. Basically, the baby needs it; if you are pregnant, now is not the time to skimp on vegetables (spinach, asparagus, romaine lettuces, beetroot, etc), enriched cereals, linseed and sunflower seeds.

8. **Vitamin B12** There is nothing better for maintaining nerve cells. But vitamin B12 also lends a hand in the production of genetic material. You will find it in milk, fish, eggs, meat and poultry.

Each to their own plateful. Man or woman, adult or child, teenager or older person, we don't all have the same **calorific needs**. Of course, things vary depending on an individual's daily energy output (the politician and the cycle courier do not exactly operate at the same tempo), but there are reliable notional figures available. Here they are, expressed as a recommended number of calories per day:

age	calories per day
child 5–9 years	1200–2100
adolescent boy	2900
adolescent girl	2500
adult male	2500
adult female*	800–2000
older male	2000-2200
older female	2100

* for pregnant women, add 100 calories in the first trimester, 200 in the second and 350 in the third

These guidelines are intended for people with a low to moderate activity level. People who move a lot obviously need more.

The 'diet' mirage

I will say it bluntly: when it comes to food, the idea of 'diet' products is one of the most successful con tricks of the modern age. You know the ones I mean: yogurts, chocolate, cartons of flavoured milk, fizzy drinks, etc. They are easy to spot thanks to the magnificent words 'Diet' or 'Slimline' or some such that probably take up half the packaging. We read the slogan and buy, persuaded that we will be able to get our figure under control by the magic of 'diet power'. What a load of cobblers! If we had food police worthy of the name, they would force the brains behind the marketing and packaging to write on their containers '0 per cent sugar, 100 per cent rip-off'.

Let's take chocolate as an example. It is made from the cocoa bean. If you don't transform it by adding sugar it remains cocoa; that is to say, a bitter inedible product. Taste some and see. So what do the manufacturers do? They replace the sugar with a sweetener and, crucially, they add more fat. And fat, just in case you missed it, is fattening. The most virtuous chocolatiers (who happen to be the most expensive) use cocoa butter. The rest opt for powdered milk, in such quantities that a product that boasts of being sugar free, or almost sugar free – but that no one has told you is actually made with fat – ends up supplying you with more calories than you would have got from eating a regular bar!

Let's not delude ourselves: there are several foods for which sugar or fat (or both) are essential ingredients. If these are reduced or cut out altogether, you're better off having something else. Take some 'diet' brioche, ice cream or biscuits. Arm yourself with a microscope (or even a telescope). Read what is written on the packaging. You are highly likely to come across an ingredient called 'glucose fructose syrup'. This compensates for the lack of regular sugar. The marketing department reassures you by explaining it is made from natural products such as wheat or corn. But they never dwell on one of its distinctive features: it increases body fat! It is also useful for bringing on diabetes and clogging up your arteries and organs. Eating too much is a sure-fire way to increase your exposure to strokes and heart attacks.

The appalling glucose fructose syrup can also be found in 'diet' yogurts, where the con trick gets even more audacious. The principle of diet yogurt? Very simple: whole milk is replaced by skimmed milk to make a product whose creamy appearance isn't exactly up to standard. Too liquid for the manufacturers' tastes (and the consumers'). The solution? Leaf gelatine. A miracle: it's now nice and creamy! This additive has no taste and no smell but its origins can be problematic: the gelatine usually comes from animal carcasses, often pigs, which Jewish and Muslim customers tend not to be aware of, unless they happen to be vegetarians. Doubtless the food industry thinks that as long as these customers don't find out, everything is fine.

The exponential growth in diet products is inversely proportional to the information made available to the consumer. The deceit has reached such heights that some neuroscientists maintain that consuming diet products makes you gain weight! They came to this conclusion by analysing the brain activity of someone drinking regular fizzy drinks (with sugar) and diet drinks (with a sugary taste but made from sweeteners).

First observation from the MRI scan: the brain's reward centre reacts differently depending on whether people drink a regular or diet drink. In the first case, it is completely satisfied. In the second, it is not: so the drinker will make up for it by eating more during his or her next meal.

The specialists' theory is founded on a simple idea: since time immemorial, the body has naturally associated energy with sweet tastes. Someone who drinks a regular fizzy drink is providing this sweet taste and energy in the form of calories the body can use. So the brain is happy. Someone who drinks a diet drink is certainly providing the sweet taste, but not the calories. The body is disappointed and, it is thought, more likely to demand extra next time we sit down for a meal, encouraging us to eat more than usual. And so to take on more calories than we need.

Of course, there are studies that say the opposite. But they are often financed by manufacturers who are making a tidy sum from sweeteners. Draw what conclusions you will . . .

To sum up, remember that 'diet' food and drink does not make you lose weight. It could even make you put on weight . . . It's an invention that enables the giants of the food-processing industry, under the pretext of taking care of your weight and health, to offer the same product in several forms for marketing reasons: a brand that exists in two forms (regular and diet) will always take up more space on supermarket shelves than a single version. I even know one brown fizzy drink that comes in regular (red packaging), diet (grey packaging), 'zero' (black packaging) and 'life' (green packaging). Four products instead of one! All the better for capturing the consumer's attention. And all the better for making nice juicy profits.

The hidden face of organic food

For some years now, we have been going organic. This is no passing fad. It is a necessary response to people having the good sense to want to protect themselves from junk food. Produce that comes from organic farms will always contain less fertilizer and fewer pesticides than food grown by conventional means, which manufacturers have been using ever since they took control of the contents of our plates. Organic products are also better than conventional ones in terms of their iron, magnesium, antioxidant and vitamin C content, particularly when it comes to potatoes. In short, all things organic are being celebrated and everyone is scrambling to get their hands on products that are labelled organic. They little suspect that one or two details are being glossed over. I would like to take a closer look at these here.

The word organic is certainly reassuring, particularly when accompanied with the Euro Leaf, the European Union's very own organic logo. And herein lies the problem. Official organic requirements are less stringent than you might imagine. In some cases, organic status is granted to products that one can find plenty to quibble about.

Whose fault is this? The supermarkets . . . Noticing the success of organic products, and enticed by the profits to be made, they pounced. With Brussels' blessing, they set about producing more to supply more, even if it meant ditching some of organic farming's fundamental principles. So livestock farms got bigger, increasing sanitary risks. Products began to be imported whose traceability was problematic. 'Organic ham' appeared in shops without anyone having spent much time looking into the conditions in which it had been prepared. Oh, it's just a minor detail, the ham is cooked with salt mixed with sodium nitrate to make sure it stays nice and pink, because that is the colour the customer is most comfortable with. Concession after concession was made to the mass-producers of organic products. Organic food is not only about creating a culture free from chemical products, it's about ethical eating too. And in this department, the processed-food industry is not always (understatement) at the cutting edge of social progress. In southern Spain, you would be sad to observe the living and working conditions of the men and women from eastern Europe who are paid a pittance to pick nice red tomatoes, green cucumbers and succulent strawberries for our supermarkets' organic ranges.

Some organic foodies, anxious not to betray their original principles, have created their own labels that you would do well to look into. It's also getting easier to find locally sourced organic food produced on a small scale. Organic is good, but it's even better when you know the provenance.

On the fringes of the crazy world of organic food, a new practice is growing: **locavorism**, or the art of 'eating local'. The term was coined by a Californian woman around ten years ago. Her name: Jessica Prentice. Her obsession: eating things that are produced less than 100 miles from her home. By doing so, she reduces her carbon footprint, enjoys fresh seasonal fruit and vegetables and forges a special bond with the farmers who supply her.

2

Good habits

Trapped by TV dinners

Ah, the TV dinner! An institution . . . Particularly for people who are in the habit of eating solo. Whereas some institutions are forces for good and command our respect (school, the Académie Française, the United Nations . . .), others deserve to be called into question. And I am only too happy to oblige.

A TV dinner involves two things: dinner and a TV (I take it we agree so far). Well, it's one thing too many . . .

Be aware: in front of the telly, everyone tends to reduce chewing and eat more quickly. It happens automatically. By failing to take your time over the task at hand – namely, eating – you are in danger of stuffing yourself silly. It takes about twenty minutes for your stomach to inform your brain that your body has had enough to eat. So, the less time you take to eat, the less time your body has to sound the alert.

What's more, your eyes are the first to stimulate your saliva glands (remember Pavlov's dog: he salivated when he saw the meat). If your eyes are glued to the flat screen they cannot fulfil their brief. Basically, if you aren't concentrating on what you are doing, your digestive system (more than capable of holding a grudge) will take great delight in letting you know it at the earliest opportunity.

TV dinners consist of watching and eating. Sooner or later you have to choose: such is life. Watch. Or eat. Watch then eat. Eat then watch. Rearrange the order however you like – just don't do both at the same time.

Breakfast: dare to eat protein!

I can never say this enough: breakfast is probably the most important meal of the day. Unless you enjoyed a feast of gargantuan proportions the night before, it is perfectly normal to get out of bed feeling peckish. The trouble is, there are some mornings when, between the high-octane wake-up and the turbo-charged exit, we grab a shower and drop 'brekkie' altogether, the whole routine lasting 15 minutes. Thinking it might help them lose weight, some people even do this on purpose, getting the wrong end of the stick – instead of the right end of a croissant. Because a croissant would be the lesser of two evils: if we are going to indulge (pastries, jam, bacon), we're better off doing so in the morning, when we have all day to burn it off, than in the evening, when we sleep and stock up.

However, you can also resolve to forego the typical French breakfast, whose combo of jam, butter, bread and croissants amounts to a festival of quick-release sugars and fats. Can you spot the mistake? Or rather, can you spot the protein? There is rarely any on our kitchen tables in the mornings. And that's a pity, because protein is our body's essential fuel. It is designed to see us through until lunchtime (which should be a light meal), without us feeling peckish at 11am. Don't hesitate to try new things: chicken or turkey breast, eggs (in all their forms) and fromage frais (with as little sugar as possible) would give you a varied, copious and above all balanced meal first thing in the morning, provided you add a bit of fruit for fibre. Addicts can wash the lot down with a tea or coffee.

One final piece of advice that just might sweep away the rest: never force yourself to eat if you aren't hungry. If that applies to you in the mornings, sorry, perhaps I should have said this at the start . . .

Avoid weight gain

There are plenty of ways to slim down and a host of experts harp on about them with dogged determination, eating a balanced diet and doing a modicum of exercise being just two. But there are also plenty of things *not to do*. Many a superfluous kilo is down to bad habits that have become entrenched in our daily routine.

Eating just before you go to bed is a terrible idea. First, because the need to do so rarely stems from hunger; it's more likely to be a sign of anxiety of some sort. Secondly, people tend to have a preference for sweet things, and calories often come with them.

Denouncing sugar does not mean you make up for it with excess salt. Though that's exactly what people do. We sometimes have a tendency to over-salt our meals, which affects blood pressure and increases water retention. It all shows up on the scales in the end.

Another habit to get out of: express-train eating. This is not an attack on the SNCF, France's honourable railway company (though I could say a few things about the price of their soggy toasted sandwiches), or any other train company for that matter, but rather a criticism of the speed at which we put our food away. Eating in less than twenty minutes is lunacy. You have to take the time to chew in order to feel full up. The brain needs time to register what you have eaten. The sooner we feel sated, the less we eat and the less weight we gain. Besides, a meal, whatever it is, deserves our full attention: we need to know how to resist the tyrannical demands of modern life that prompt us to do other things while we eat (watching TV, playing with our mobile phone). These bad habits distract us from the task at hand and trick us into eating more than we need to.

Then there's what happens between meals: we don't drink enough water and that encourages fluid retention. It means our kidneys work in slow motion and fail to expel enough of the waste products that pollute our bodies.

So, to recap: eating salty food, quickly, while doing something else entirely, just before bed, having failed to drink enough water beforehand gives you a clean sweep of the Top Five things to ban. Cutting out one or several of these will stop you putting on weight.

What is a portion?

The notion of portion size is vague to say the least. How big is a portion? How do you measure it? Should you weigh your food? No: all you need are your hands and a plate.

A portion of fruit can be measured by making a fist. Eating strawberries? Help yourself to a volume that corresponds more or less to the size of your fist. An apple? That ought to do it. A pear? Yup. Mandarins? Two of them will make a portion.

Now, unclench your fist and bring your two hands together to make a scoop. Fill that with vegetables and you have your portion (but be a bit stingier if you're going for sweetcorn, peas or potatoes).

Fancy a piece of cheese? Go ahead. Point your index and middle fingers, bring them together and you've got a portion size.

Some meat, poultry or fish? Open your hand and serve yourself an amount that corresponds to the size of your palm.

If you need to transpose this trick to a plateful, use the magic 'four quarters' rule. Put a plate in front of you. Divide it into four (mentally). You now have four quarters (primary school maths). The portion of meat should take up one quarter of the plate. The starch should take up another quarter. And the two last quarters (therefore half of the plate) will be left for vegetables.

Place a yogurt and a portion of fruit next to the plate and you are ready to eat a balanced meal.

The art of digestion

I will never say it too often: good digestion stems from a healthy and balanced diet. But that isn't enough: you should also adopt a few habits to relieve your stomach and aid the digestive process.

You have doubtless noticed that you have teeth. Thirty-two, to be precise. Dentists will confirm this . . . The trick is to use them. Avoiding too many soft foods (such as yogurts and squidgy bread) and opting for things that you have to grind up will get your teeth working. Chew. Chew again. Keep chewing. Chew lots, chew more! Food that has been reduced to a pulp and mixed with the enzymes in your saliva will be given a right royal welcome by your body. You just need to be aware of this and take your time when you sit down to eat. Believe me: eating your lunch or evening meal in five minutes flat is an act of war on your tum and, sooner or later, it will take its revenge.

Another thing: do you drink water? You don't? You need to get to it, urgently. You will? Excellent. But be advised: down those bottles *between* rather than during meals. A glass with a meal is good. But too much water with food will impair digestion by interfering with the enzymes' work.

Lastly, make fruit count. As I may have mentioned once or twice, it is good for you. Some people recommend eating it between meals, others doubt whether this advice is remotely scientific (see the entry on p.156) but remember the most salient point: you must not go without.

Be alcohol intelligent

Alcohol accounts for 45,000 deaths a year in France. It is the second highest avoidable cause of death after tobacco, is connected to many road and workplace accidents and, over time, gives rise to a raft of pathologies including cancer (mouth, throat, intestinal, liver), heart disease, high blood pressure, cirrhosis of the liver . . . I think I'll stop there, so as not to spoil the small glass you enjoy from time to time. I am, of course, referring to that major public health problem: *excessive* alcohol consumption.

I emphasize 'excessive' because I don't want to give the impression that I have got it in for alcohol consumption in general, which, in a country like France, would be taking the double risk of antagonizing a whole industrial sector and coming across as the biggest killjoy ever. I am the first to admit that having a glass of something is very pleasant but in this, as in everything, I recommend moderation and information. Drink, but do it intelligently.

Drinking intelligently means, first of all, not drinking on an empty stomach. It's essential to eat before you drink, since food reduces the speed at which alcohol passes into the bloodstream. This takes thirty minutes on an empty stomach and an hour when you drink with food.

Drinking intelligently means taking the time to taste and relish your drink. Taking one's time, a notion I champion throughout this book, is a way of pinpointing what we like or don't like drinking. In general, the first sip sparks an explosion of smells and tastes. The sips that follow are less intense but also less flavourful until, eventually, they are stripped of all appeal. You must be on the lookout for the precise moment your taste buds become saturated. And deduce that it's time to stop drinking.

Drinking intelligently means limiting yourself to your favourite alcoholic drinks. Some are more agreeable than others: accept the ones you enjoy, turn down the others.

Drinking intelligently also means knowing how to say no. It is essential to invoke your freedom to drink or *not* to drink. That way you avoid letting yourself be influenced by group or peer pressure, and you ignore those who say annoying things like: 'People who don't drink don't like having fun.'

Drinking intelligently means being aware of what is going on in the body from the first sip. Alcohol is absorbed by the wall of the small intestine and passes into the bloodstream. In a matter of minutes it is conveyed around the whole body, and to one organ in particular, the brain, before being expelled. Only 5 per cent is excreted by the kidneys (in the form of urine), the skin (sweat), the lungs (exhaled air) and saliva. The liver deals with the rest. Up to 95 per cent of alcohol expulsion is undertaken by the liver. We owe it a lot: it acts like a tiny water purification plant, cleansing the blood of the alcohol it contains (just one of its five hundred essential duties). If you overindulge, it will let you know in its own way: in extreme cases, alcohol can be responsible for hepatitis (inflammation of the liver) or liver cancer.

Lastly, drinking intelligently means spreading out alcoholic drinks over the course of a meal and the days of the week. The calorific value of alcohol is far from negligible: if your intake is too high in relation to your body's needs, you will begin to store those calories. And storing means weight gain! Particularly because once a molecule of alcohol has been transformed by the body it actually increases the likelihood of storing fatty and sugary foods, thanks to a chemical reaction whose complexity I shall spare you.

Alcohol and calories

The size of the drink may vary, but no single alcoholic drink is particularly less calorific than the rest: 3cl of whisky, 12cl of wine, a glass of champagne and half a litre of beer all come with roughly the same number of calories – somewhere between 80 and 210:

- a 12cl glass of wine contains around 100 calories
- a half-litre of beer 140 calories
- a glass of champagne between 80 and 120 calories
- a martini 210 calories!

I'm not talking about cocktails, where fruit juice, cane sugar and coconut milk are added to make one big calorie factory. If such blends are to your taste, try to mix alcohol with 100 per cent pure fruit and vegetable juices, rather than fizzy or flavoured drinks. These are of low nutritional value and are often made with sweeteners. When mixed with an artificially sweetened drink, alcohol passes into the bloodstream more quickly and the blood alcohol content skyrockets.

Alcohol is a liar

'Rethink your third drink.' 'Don't drown your future.' For decades, admen have pushed their creativity to the limit, making an impact (and quite a lot of money) with memorable slogans that alert us to the dangers of alcohol abuse. I have no doubt my approach will be less engaging but it will be more scientific and more useful. That said, I'm equally capable of giving in to the slogan fad. I would go for something like: 'Alcohol is lying to you.'

Who has never succumbed to the euphoria of champagne? Who has never enjoyed the feeling of well-being that comes over you, that makes you laugh out loud and talk with brio, when there's a glass in your hand? Watch out: alcohol is lying to you. Drinks with fizz contain carbon dioxide and cause alcohol blood content to increase more quickly. The bubbles are thought to make it easier for alcohol to pass into the bloodstream. What's more, they speed up the emptying of the stomach and it is likely this leads to alcohol being absorbed even more quickly in the small intestine.

As you can see, there is a lot going on in your (new-found) dream body when the booze (champagne or other) is flowing.

And things are also happening up in the cortex: you become disinhibited, you feel invincible, when really you are more vulnerable than ever.

Yes, alcohol is lying to you. While you're giggling, it is quietly going to work on your central nervous system. So as not to dramatically increase the effects, and because of the potential dangers involved, you shouldn't combine alcohol with other psychoactive substances, including anxiety-reducing medicines or drugs such as cannabis (whose use, may I remind any amnesiacs, is theoretically illegal, alcohol or no alcohol). There is a synergy between these substances and alcohol; their combined depressive effects are greater than the sum of their parts.

Yes, alcohol lies to you. It creeps up in disguise, spun by talented marketing people and concealed in flavoured beers or so-called fusion drinks (grapefruit rosés or peach white wines, for example), which go down a treat on café terraces and at a party. These supposedly classy beverages are enjoying more and more success. A nice colour, chilled, a pleasant taste without bitterness, they slip down so easily: these drinks have a knack of making people forget they contain alcohol. We drink, then we drink a bit more: well, it's not doing much, right? But they have exactly the same side effects in store for you as any other form of alcohol.

You've been drinking, you feel good, you feel warm, you strip off . . . Watch out: alcohol is lying to you. Never forget that the feelings it gives you are deceptive. The warmth that comes over you, glass in hand, is merely due to the dilation of the blood vessels beneath the skin. All alcohol does is displace internal heat, bringing it to the body's surface.

You're still feeling good, so you treat yourself to 'one last glass' for the umpteenth time. You feel even warmer now. Why not have a cigarette? Alcohol greatly increases the desire to smoke. After all, culturally, the two practices are strongly associated. You don't feel it, but your body is suffering. Silently. It keeps it to itself. It too is lying to you. By omission. Under the influence. Because while you're chuckling happily, your kidneys are working flat out and your liver is going full pelt. Expelling alcohol is a big ask for the kidneys. They need water to do this. As a result, you become dehydrated. Ah, all this liquid! Does the act of drinking and the fact you don't feel thirsty make you think you are hydrating yourself? Quite the reverse. But how are you supposed to know, when alcohol is lying to you? Meanwhile, your liver is busy metabolizing the ethanol. To do so, it turns it into acetaldehyde and this is when things can turn ugly. You see, this substance causes nausea, vomiting, sweating . . . You've overdone it, time to pay. And the bill will seem all the steeper because, when dehydrated, the body is subjected to generalized stress.

Now come the regrets ('I shouldn't have') and the resolutions ('I *will* limit myself to four units of alcohol at any one time'), a bout of excessive consumption having led to drunkenness and severe alcoholic intoxication. The body is poisoned.

Alcohol, that big fat liar, has another fault: no sense of fairness. Women and men are not equal in the face of this deceit. Assuming the same amount is consumed, the ladies are more susceptible to its effects than you are, gentlemen. It is a biological fact. And gender is not the only factor that influences blood alcohol elimination. To have a better understanding of how the effects of alcohol and toxicity can vary, you need to consider body size, age and genetic background (see p. 61). On that note, 'cheers', but 'cheers' in moderation . . .

Genes and alcohol Some good news: alcoholism is not a genetically transmitted disease. Although, as is often the case, things are actually more nuanced than that, and there *are* genes that are linked to addictive behaviours in general. So if a father suffers from alcohol dependency, his children are more at risk of becoming alcoholics themselves. However, the sons and daughters of alcoholics are often lifetime teetotallers who don't drink alcohol at all because they have had to endure the effects it had on their parents' behaviour.

Reducing your alcohol consumption

There are a great many people who, while not considering themselves alcoholics, have let alcohol take hold in the name of conviviality or by force of habit. Surreptitiously. Knocking back a glass at the slightest opportunity has become a habit and it has made them social alcoholics, oblivious to what is happening: they are in the last stage of the descent to full-blown alcoholism. Awareness is a prerequisite of action. And taking action consists of doing little things that need to be done, adopting little habits that need to be adopted, asking little questions that need to be asked. Do not take these changes lightly: they may seem slight but they are an immense help.

Have you ever asked yourself what makes you drink? What triggers your desire? From stress at work to a yearning to overcome one's shyness, there are a thousand (arguable) pretexts. Identify them and it will be easier for you to avoid repeatedly finding yourself in situations where drinking alcohol seems the right thing to do.

Have you asked yourself what reasons there might be for wanting to cut down your consumption? Have a think and you are bound to find some, and they might well go beyond the obvious positive consequences for your health and well-being. You must start here if this approach is to be effective. What do you want? To have more energy? To control bouts of anger? To improve your relationships with other people? To sleep better? To look after your skin? To be a good role model? Based on our own lifestyle, every one of us is capable of answering questions such as these. Provided we want to take the time to ask them . . .

People who know how to appreciate alcohol without becoming slaves to it employ little tricks that they have found effective. When you have a drink, take the time to enjoy it, make the pleasure last, take a sip and keep it in your mouth long enough to savour it. Follow the example of sommeliers; they love wine and they know how to drink.

And why not try 'slow drinking'? Specifically, taking small sips and putting your glass down between each one. Yes, putting it down. It might seem a silly thing to say, but putting your glass down more frequently is a very good way of drinking less from it. And if your glass empties more slowly, your blood alcohol level will rise more slowly. Obvious, isn't it? Child's play really. Yes, but it works. And when someone is offering to buy the next round it's easier to resist if your glass is still full.

You can also set yourself challenges. If you find yourself drinking every day out of habit, you can reduce your consumption by picking one or maybe even two dry days a week. A third will be appreciably easier, and triply appreciated by your body! Mind you, you mustn't make up for the 24 or 48 hours of abstinence by drinking more on the other days . . .

Try, as far as is possible, to push drinking your first glass to later on in the day. For example, don't have a drink with lunch, particularly if it's hot weather. Don't forget, alcohol dehydrates you.

Don't mix several types of alcoholic drink in one evening, so do not succumb to the classic sequence of aperitif + white wine + red wine + digestif. Choose one drink and stick to it.

Be systematic about your alcohol consumption: when you know you are going to drink, decide in advance the maximum number of glasses you will allow yourself in an evening. Ideally make it fewer than four, assuming you're not driving of course.

Finally, if you want to reduce the amount you drink, let people know about it. Inform your friends and family. Ask them, directly, to help you stay true to your word. And if they feel like passing comment, don't take it the wrong way. They love you really . . .

One too many

Who can boast of being immune to veisalgia? (Make a note: 'veisalgia' is the medical term for a hangover.) So who can? Not many people. Not even me, I mean . . . Ahem . . . The thing is, even if one has a reputation for being sober, it only takes one little *soirée* – two flutes and three glasses, say – to wake up the next morning wearing a German helmet with the spike on the inside, as the French say. The most important thing is that it doesn't happen too regularly. When it does, it's useful to know some tricks for coming out the other side.

Woozy? Nauseous? Dry mouth? Head like a drum? Want to

die? Start by drinking water. I'll say that again: water. When you drink alcohol you make your kidneys work harder than they should. To expel the alcohol they use water. And do you know where they find it? Not in the fountain at the corner of the street, but in your body. The logical consequence: you become dehydrated. Hence the need to drink more than usual. From the tap or a bottle, there is nothing better than water to get yourself up and about. I recommend one glass for every two glasses of alcohol consumed. Any other drink will just complicate matters. Coffee, with its diuretic effect, will dehydrate you even more and raise your heart rate. As for juice, orange or grapefruit are both likely to be too acidic for you to handle.

Then, eat! Yes, eat. The morning after, we sometimes feel like we can't swallow a thing. Mistake: you have to force yourself. But hang on: that doesn't mean I'm giving you carte blanche to finish the peanuts and the creamy pudding from the night before. Shun fat and go for a few boiled vegetables instead, to give your liver and stomach a rest, because they have been boozing as well . . .

Failing that, there is one method for dealing with a hangover that is infallible and irrefutable, a tried and tested sure-fire winner handed down from generation to generation (and it won't cost you a penny): avoid having one in the first place. How? Give your drinking arm a rest. The choice is yours . . .

Your fridge is a germ factory

Can you imagine living without your fridge? Of course you can't. It's part of the furniture, figuratively if not quite literally, and vital to our way of life. But do you treat it right? Do you really look after it and therefore, indirectly, yourself?

I should explain.

It cannot have escaped your attention that the fridge contains a stack of things that end up, sooner or later, inside your body. You have to be vigilant with food. A badly maintained fridge can turn into a germ factory. But germs can't survive the cold, I hear you say. Wrong! With their strong little biceps they build defences and learn to withstand low temperatures.

So it is crucial your fridge is cleaned twice a month. At least. Don't use household products, certainly not bleach: you could end up tasting it on your food. Instead, just sponge it down with alcohol vinegar, dry it with a soft cloth and Bob's your uncle. Then fill it up again, being sure to cover any opened products carefully. Owning a fridge requires elbow grease!

Clean up the ambient air

I'm sure you're fond of your home. It's important to live in pleasant surroundings, in a place that reflects who you are and makes you feel good, particularly during the winter months when we're only too happy to spend more time indoors.

You do need to clean the air you breathe because, what with humidity, mildew, flooring, upholstery, motorized vehicles (I could go on), sooner or later you are going to expose yourself to allergies, irritations and headaches.

The first thing to do is air your home. Whether it's raining, blowing a gale, snowing or gloriously sunny, and regardless of the temperature outside, you must never forget the simple act of opening windows. A few minutes every day will suffice but it is essential for depolluting air that is going to wind up in your lungs.

As well as getting into the habit of airing your home, you can also try using essential oils. You're better off buying these from aromatherapy experts in specialized shops, rather than going online, as they need to be transported quite carefully. Lavender, rosemary, eucalyptus, thyme, grapefruit or pine all help purify and aromatize the ambient air. Their antibacterial and antiviral properties increase your chances of gliding healthily from one season to the next. And they will help you breathe better. To diffuse them (always cold), use a nebulizer for 15 minutes in a bedroom and half an hour in a living room. This is always healthier than using candles, many of which emit fumes and pollute more than they purify.

> To chase away those little smells that get up your nose (and on your nerves) you have an ally: **bicarbonate of soda**. Put two dessert spoons in a cup or a small bowl and let it work its magic. Nasty smells will be absorbed.

Operation Clean Hands

It is the simplest thing in the world, but 95 per cent of people do it badly, or only half do it. Yes, 95 per cent! What is it? I warn you, this will blow your socks off: 95 per cent of people don't know how to wash their hands properly.

Oh, come on . . . Is there really a technique to hand washing? An art to scrubbing? A secret to soaping? And, nine out of ten people don't know what it is? Apparently, yes. That, at any rate, is the conclusion reached by respected researchers from the equally respected University of Michigan (who lambast men in particular, by the way).

We know that Americans have a habit of overdramatizing. We also know that stark warnings are good but gentle advice is better. So, here we go . . .

Washing your hands is not just a matter of rinsing them with water. You have to soap them, properly soap them: a minimum of 20 seconds is recommended for comprehensive hygiene.

Nor is washing your hands about washing *just* your hands. You have to remember your wrists if you're serious about destroying all trace of germs. You also need to be precise, bordering on fanatical. Make sure you rub between the fingers and give the palms special attention. That is what it takes to get rid of all the bacteria that relish lurking there.

There are hundreds of good reasons for remembering to wash your hands several times a day (particularly in the evening when you are more relaxed and so more inclined to go with the flow). It is non-negotiable after going to the toilet (sorry to spell it out, but it seems that this obvious point still eludes some people), and should also be done after using public transport, blowing your nose, using door handles, playing with your mobile phone and driving. And *before* cooking and sitting down to eat.

As I'm sure you've realized, it's not about having clean hands for the sake of it; we all make a habit of touching our face, and our mouth, eyes and nose are splendid entry points for germs. Good hygiene helps limit, or even eliminate, the spread of viruses and infections, especially in wintertime. Washing your hands is the main way to avoid catching a cold. This advice applies to everyone but is especially important for children; they are particularly vulnerable under the age of six as their immune systems are not fully developed.

Caffeine: go easy if you're pregnant

You like coffee. You drink it regularly. I don't blame you, it's very nice. But if you're pregnant, some things have got to change.

The good news, contrary to a view doing the rounds, is that you don't have to quit completely, just moderate your consumption: an absolute maximum of two – oh, all right, three – cups a day. I'm nice like that.

The reason is simple. Coffee contains caffeine. It is a stimulant. And a pregnant woman needs calm.

But that's not all. The French National Institute for Health and Medical Research had the bright idea of giving caffeine to mice. They concluded that it was harmful to the foetal development of Mickey and Minnie Mouse. It made them more susceptible to epileptic seizures.

Now, it hasn't escaped my attention that you are not a mouse but a woman. A particularly resplendent woman getting ready to bring a new person into the world. However, it is more than likely that what doesn't suit rodents doesn't suit you either. Better to be safe than sorry.

One last thing: it's not the coffee that's questionable but the caffeine. Caffeine is also found in tea. So limit yourself to one or two cups a day. It's also in some fizzy drinks, including a very famous one that starts with Coca and ends with Cola. Consume them sensibly, especially because they aren't very good for the waistline either. Yours is expanding for the *right* reasons at the moment; you don't need any help from that stuff.

Moisturizing creams: the essential and the scandalous

When it rains, you put on a hat and scarf and wrap yourself up as much as possible, layer upon layer, but, come what may, your face will be out in the open. So it's a good idea to protect it by taking care of your skin.

How? Here's how:

1. Think about cleansing your skin, but doing so gently. Morning and night, using thermal spring water rather than tap water. The latter tends to dry out the skin.
2. Don't skimp: get a decent moisturizer. Apply it in the morning before going out or in the evening before going to bed; it will restore elasticity to the skin on your face. Feel free to put some on your neck too.
3. As well as moisturizer, it is worth using a neutralizing skincare product. They are ideal for reducing redness caused by exposure to the elements.
4. Remember your lips. There is a plethora of moisturizing balms, made with cocoa butter, shea butter or simply 'natural', and perhaps with added vitamins (A and E). Keep a tube to hand and apply it to your lips several times a day. They are particularly prone to exposure and can become fragile in bad weather.

These words of advice might seem self-evident to anyone for whom keeping the skin permanently moisturized is the most obvious thing in the world (particularly women, who are better versed in the practice on the whole). Plenty of people would agree. Moisturizing cream is the queen of beauty products. Some 20 million French citizens regularly apply it to their faces, some to their bodies too. First observation: 20 million is good. It's actually a lot. But I was under the impression the population of France is 65 million, and that leaves a big margin for improvement. And margins – more specifically profit margins – lead me on to my second observation. You are being taken for a ride! Yes, they have conned you into believing that the more expensive a cream, the more effective it will be. Rubbish! It's a scam. Sometimes, the opposite is even true.

I'll explain. There are all sorts of creams and they come at all sorts of prices. Let's make this simple: you can find some that cost €3, some that set you back €20 and some that easily exceed €50. Those who can afford to eagerly grab the most expensive. The less fortunate tend to opt for the mid-range, telling themselves that a cream that costs less than €5 cannot be the real deal. This is how logic works in the popular subconscious: more expensive means more effective. Allow me to set the record straight: that is codswallop!

Cosmetic laboratories regularly test samples to measure skin hydration levels before and after applying cream. This is known as corneometry, the process whereby the effectiveness of a moisturizing product is evaluated. The labs regularly reach the same conclusion: there is no difference between the various creams, even though their price tags vary enormously.

To work out what's going on, have a look at the packaging, where a cream's ingredients are listed. The most expensive products unfurl an impressive list of active hydrating elements and plant extracts, positioned in a sufficiently eye-catching manner to hook you before you approach the till. An abundance of active ingredients is no guarantee of effectiveness – far from it. I advise you in the strongest terms: go for the cheap creams that make do with a few good-quality active ingredients, such as glycerine and panthenol. Remember: when it comes to moisturizers, less is more. Lots of cheap creams get straight to the heart of the matter. Yes, they have fewer active ingredients, but the ones they do have are known to work. The rest are selling a dream; the prestige of a brand with packaging galore but results that sometimes leave one feeling sceptical. Because a cream's impact boils down to how long it lasts. There's no point smearing it on your face first thing in the morning only to notice that it has lost its hydrating properties two hours later. A good cream works for a minimum of four hours. Again, in blind lab tests, some cheap creams have proved longer lasting than the famous brands. The difference in price is down to the manufacturers' and distributors' profit margins and the cost of the advertising they blitz you with in women's magazines and ad breaks on TV (of unrivalled glamour, it must be said).

Nails of steel!

You may not have noticed, but the changing of the seasons has repercussions for your nails. Yes, your nails. I could pontificate for hours about why they become fragile, but as I'm supposed to be giving simple advice here, let's cut straight to the chase: how to avoid them breaking (without recourse to varnish, which makes them brittle). Of course, this applies to men too: they're also allowed to have strong nails, and are advised that women have a habit of checking out their hands . . .

The first step is to prepare an oil bath. Olive or sweet almond, take your pick. Add a few drops of lemon juice: this will whiten your nails slightly. Now simply soak the ends of your fingers for quarter of an hour or so. Your nails will be shinier and, more importantly, better protected.

Time for step two: moisturizing. Use a hand cream. Take your time rubbing it in so the cream really penetrates. This has the added effect of softening your cuticles (the layer of skin covering the base of your nails).

Next? Zzzz . . . Just leave it to work throughout the night. By the way, there is nothing to stop you using oil instead of cream; argan or cocoa butter oil will do the job just as well.

You will soon be telling everyone about the effectiveness of this little ceremony, which should be repeated once a week. You can also take brewer's yeast for a month. It is a natural fortifier and good for nails. And hair too. So, don't hold back.

Sit properly and give your back a break

Have you noticed that back pain regularly makes the front pages of magazines? There is a reason for this: it sells. And why does it sell, do you think? Because it affects everyone. Permanently or sporadically.

I know what's to blame. I know because it sometimes makes my life a misery too. Slouching. When you round your back, your posture – which seems relaxing – becomes permanently effortful. You think you're taking it easy when really your body is gritting its teeth. And who pays for it? The back. Slouching is a scourge. It lies in wait for you the whole time, ready to pounce the moment your bottom touches a chair.

Now, during the day, for practical reasons, you're often sitting down. It's important to get into good habits, starting with these:

1. Avoid sitting for too long: limit the time you spend sitting or break it up over the day.
2. If you must sit a lot, adopt good posture and avoid being too still.

'But,' you say, 'what is good posture?' Good question . . . I was just coming to that. Good posture when working at your desk requires:

- support for your back
- your bottom to be firmly placed at the back of your chair
- your keyboard and screen to be opposite you, to avoid trunk rotation
- your forearms to rest on the desk, so the lumbar spine doesn't take their weight
- the mouse to be as close to you as possible, to avoid stretching your back to reach it
- your eyes to be at screen height and at a distance of around 50cm from it

Let me go into a bit more detail. When at your computer, you might sometimes struggle to read small characters. My advice: enlarge the font size. Never move your face closer to the screen: that will automatically lead to back rounding. And, back rounding is where the trouble starts. You have been warned.

For the more sensitive among you, it's quite a good idea to opt for an ergonomic chair, with a seat back that matches the curvature of the spine. Be sure to wedge your pelvis right back in the seat. I'll let you into a little secret: I work at my computer sitting on a Swiss ball, a large inflatable ball about 70cm in diameter, the sort you see in gyms. You can buy them in sport shops and some supermarkets. It's a way of working your core muscles without realizing you're doing it.

Your back needs exercise

Physical activity is an excellent way of preventing back pain. It improves core muscle strength, which, in turn, means your lumbar vertebrae don't have to work so hard. When we exert ourselves, in whatever way, numerous muscles in the body join forces to achieve the desired result. The wide range of activities we undertake all contribute to the body's muscle development. Having good musculature makes physical effort easier and helps us maintain good posture. It limits spinal injuries too.

The king of sports, for someone who wants to take care of their back and strengthen their back muscles, is swimming. The body floats in water. So the restrictions caused by body weight acting on the spine are taken out of the equation.

However, choose your stroke carefully: avoid butterfly, which exerts the most tension on the spine (mind you, if you're new to swimming I doubt you'll be starting with the butterfly). My advice is breaststroke. But not any old breaststroke. Use head-down breaststroke: make sure you put your head under the water with each stroke or your back will arch. Crawl is also good, but be sure to turn your head to one side and then the other. Always breathing on the same side teaches the body 'asymmetric' habits – not a good idea. Then there's back crawl, ideal for beating back pain. But more physically demanding and not great if you want to avoid getting splashed in the face, or worse.

So, I have given you these glowing recommendations, and now come the objections: I don't like the water, I can't swim, the pool is too far away, etc. Okay, I get it. But, I'm not beaten yet. Do you know that using an exercise bike develops your back muscles? Do you know that mastering the art of the mini-dumb-bell workout develops your back muscles? Do you know that yoga develops your back muscles? Do you know that walking develops your back muscles? Do you know that you've run out of excuses? Move! Move at your own rhythm, play sport or do any form of exercise that appeals to you, but move. The simple act of stretching, making yourself more flexible, gardening or choosing to walk to the shops rather than take the car will be beneficial to you. Make a note: your back's worst enemy is inactivity.

Little everyday movements that wreck your back

Every day, a hundred and one situations put strain on our bodies without us even noticing. And then one day, *crunch*: you've got backache. You know the saying: prevention is the best medicine. That means it's better to get into good habits as soon as you can, and turn them into learned patterns of behaviour. This will stop you yodelling in pain when it's too late.

Let's take the car as an example. We can spend hours in it, sometimes feeling impatient and stressed. 'I must be relaxed,' we tell ourselves, so we tilt back the seat for more comfort. Mistake. In the car, you should adjust the seat to make it upright and make sure the steering wheel isn't too far away. It is vital to drive with the upper body in contact with the back of the car seat. You can wedge a cushion against your lower back if need be. If the seat is too hard, and you're feeling every vibration and jolt, place another cushion beneath you. I realize that's a lot of cushions, and it may not be very stylish, but your back is worth it.

Paradoxically, resting can also be pretty deadly. Starting with the super-duper sofa you love to sprawl out on, making the most of its comfy softness. It cost you an arm and a leg, I expect. Well, it could cost you a back as well! It is highly likely you lounge with poor posture, stretching your legs out in front of you and resting them on the coffee table. You feel like you're relaxing but in fact you're storing up pain for another day. In this position, the squashed vertebrae risk trapping a nerve and that can lead to inflammation and muscle spasms. Be warned: anything that causes you to round your lower back is bad. From now on, when you're enjoying the comforts of your sitting room, reading or surfing on a screen of some sort, consider placing a cushion against your lower back, another one under your neck and a third under your knees.

Generally, it's important for your spine to stay vertical. Since we always favour the easy option, we forget this, particularly when carrying a heavy object or bending down (or rather bending *over*) to pick something up off the ground. Again, bad move. Think vertical.

If the spinal column is vertical when effort is exerted, the weight is spread evenly over the intervertebral discs. They act like shock-absorbing rings between the rigid vertebrae. They can withstand a great deal of pressure and your spine won't be in danger. If, on the other hand, some parts of your spine are not vertical, pressure is concentrated on one part of the disc only: the pressure can be five to ten times higher at this spot than across the rest of the disc. The disc tends to slip to the side where there is less pressure. And, guess what, your body isn't stupid; in fact it's pretty clever: it detects this extreme pressure on one area of the disc and, reacting to the danger, contracts the whole of the affected area. Consequence: a good bout of lumbago, as the back rapidly stiffens due to a muscle contraction that occurs while exerting effort with bad posture.

I can hear some people chuckling sceptically and saying to themselves: 'I've been getting on fine for years without being obsessed with keeping my spine vertical.' They are wrong. The body compensates. The body regulates. The body supports. But if too much is asked of it, one day it will crack . . .

Little daily exercises to combat back pain

Here are some exercises to help improve your posture and pelvic mobility, and relieve back problems:

- Stand up and hollow out the base of your back. Your pelvis is now tipped forward (or anteverted). Next, tip it backwards by rounding your lower back (it is now retroverted). Repeat this movement, but be sure to stay upright; your torso shouldn't move. Being more aware of the position of your pelvis should help you instinctively hold it in the retroverted position, which helps relax the lower back muscles.

- Another way to ease back tension is to stand upright with your back against a wall, extend your arms upwards and try to make yourself as tall as you can, without lifting your heels off the floor. Keep your chin level while extending your head upwards. In this position, you are stretching out your back muscles, which should offer some relief. Hold the position for about 10 seconds, remembering to breathe deeply.

- Lower back pain can also be caused by weak abdominal and back muscles. Tone your abs with regular exercises and find some core-strengthening exercises to help support the back muscles. Don't neglect your glutes (bum muscles) and hamstrings (at the back of the thighs). Stretch these carefully when you feel they need it, avoiding sudden movements.

An eye-watering number of screens

With the advent of the technological age, the computer has become man's best friend. And woman's. The screen, simultaneously workplace tool and leisure companion, commands our attention: when we are in front of one, whether writing or reading, we concentrate.

Consequence: we blink less.

Consequence of the consequence: our pupils are less lubricated and the lachrymal film is broken, which gives us dry eyes.

Consequence of the consequence of the consequence: fatigue, stinging eyes, redness, all sorts of unpleasant stuff, basically.

To remedy this, the best thing to do is have a good cry. Still, I'd rather you didn't lose that famous smiley disposition of yours, so here is something else to try: force yourself to blink. Even if you don't feel the need. You can also use eyewash: artificial tears offer some relief.

As well as this practical measure, you should watch your diet, so your body has all it needs to make tears easily. It's another reason to pick foods that are known to contain omega-3s and antioxidants.

Finally, you can also decide to spend less time in front of the computer. That, we all know, is easier said than done. But there is nothing to stop you trying . . .

Yes to dark glasses, but only if they are good quality

ARMD. Ring a bell? This acronym stands for Age-Related Macular Degeneration, which, along with cataracts, can become your worst enemy if you don't protect your eyes from the sun. I'm sure you own a pair of sunglasses. I'm equally sure they look amazing on you. But are they the right ones for you? Read on to find out, and tell yourself that making great savings is *not* the priority here.

1. **The frames** Ideally, they should wrap around the contour of your eyebrows so as to provide as much coverage as possible. Wide arms prevent light sneaking in at the sides.
2. **The lens material** The job of the lenses is to form a barrier against ultraviolet rays. They can be polycarbonate (the most efficient), CR 39 resin, or mineral lenses; it doesn't matter. The main thing is that they conform to European standards (look for the CE marking). Remember: the clearer the lens, the less protection it offers from glare.
3. **The class of lens** This determines the amount of light that reaches the retina. The scale goes from zero to four and any self-respecting seller will make sure it's clearly labelled on the glasses. Class 1? Run a mile. Class 2? Fine, but not amazing. Class 3? The one I recommend, and the most widely available. Class 4? Mostly reserved for children over six months. Or designed for mountain sports, where the brightness is intense. But don't wear a pair at the wheel. You have to choose, it's seeing or driving – everyone knows that.

Suncream, instructions for use

No sun without suncream! Don't play games with your skin or you might get burnt. It hurts, for one thing, but more importantly a lifetime of repeated sunburn can add up to a malignant melanoma, the sophisticated term for skin cancer.

Of course, you want to tan. And tan quickly. So it's very tempting to use a low-factor cream. Hideous mistake: go for factor 30 (minimum) and consider going up to 50 if you have fair skin.

Applying suncream is tedious. You have to fight the temptation to do a rushed job. Mistake number two: if you look like a piece of buttered toast you are not protected. You should carefully spread the cream over your body and make sure you really rub it into the skin. Sounds fastidious? It is. Just think of the good time you are about to have in the sun. Ideally you turn the 'buttering' into a ritual that is performed at home, before going out. Put it everywhere, including on your toes. And top up regularly. Don't wait until you feel yourself starting to burn.

A mistake to avoid: leaving your **skin-protection products** lying around in the sun for hours. Cosmetics do not like extreme temperatures. Leave your creams in the shade of a bag, where they will be protected from high temperatures.

Flip or flop?

Ah, flip flops. They have staged something of a comeback over the last few years. They are worthy of national debate or, failing that, a quick appraisal here: 'for or against'?

For: they are easy to put on and take off and you know they will keep your feet aired when it's really hot.

Against: we might love flip flops but wearing them all the time can damage the feet:

1. Flip flops make your toes work. You have to 'grip' so your foot doesn't slip out. I suppose it's a workout of sorts, but if you're constantly asking your muscles to work in this way it can lead to tendonitis, i.e. inflammation of the tendons.
2. The sole of flip flops being what it is (thin, very thin), the foot absorbs considerable impact with each step. Long term, you run the risk of causing hairline fractures of the foot bones.
3. When walking in flip flops your bare skin rubs against plastic, a bonanza for bacteria. This can also can cause blisters.

That said, I'm fairly sure flip flops don't threaten the future of the human race. I would simply say, if you like wearing them, choose carefully: pick a style that isn't too soft (if you can bend them in half, forget it), go for thick soles, don't discount the soft-leather version and tell yourself that flip flops are a perishable product and need replacing every year.

Avoid swimmer's ear

Scandalmongers sometimes claim that French doctors who work over the summer love *otitis externa*, because it's a nice little earner. Swimmer's ear . . . In fine weather, sufferers pitch up in doctors' waiting rooms by the lorryload. Those who have experienced it will tell you it can ruin a good chunk of your summer holidays.

What is swimmer's ear? It all starts with water (from the sea, a lake, a swimming pool or even the bath, there is opportunity aplenty) accumulating in the outer ear. There, bacteria and fungi say to themselves: 'This is great! Let's run riot!' Then they run riot. And you cop it . . . Need a diagnosis? Delicately pull your ear upwards. Does it hurt? In that case, it's swimmer's ear. Time to make an appointment with a doctor and kiss swimming goodbye.

So, to avoid spoiling your fun, here is my advice:

1. **Don't use cotton buds in the ear canal,** particularly if you don't know how to use them properly. You are in danger of stockpiling cerumen (otherwise known as earwax) and that is not the aim of the exercise.
2. **Tip your head to each side after swimming** With a bit of luck and perseverance the trapped water will trickle out. Then dab your ear dry with the corner of a clean towel or a tissue. If water stays trapped for a while, you have got a wax blockage. You see, cerumen is hydrophilic and expands upon contact with water.
3. **Swim in clean waters,** where possible, and avoid putting your head under. I hear you: asking children not to put their heads underwater is tantamount to putting the fox in the henhouse with strict instructions to eat only the grain. It ain't going to

happen . . . So, on to the ultimate solution (that you can use too because it is just as effective for adults): special ear plugs for swimming. With these, your progeny can frolic in (relative) peace.

Look after your décolleté

There is a subject, ladies, that concerns you as much as it fascinates men: your cleavage. As a woman, there is every chance you care about yours. And quite right too. It's certainly worth protecting the skin of the cleavage. This area of the body, where there is a paucity of sebaceous glands (they secrete sebum that prevents the skin from drying out), is delicate, not to say fragile. There is a danger of the skin ageing prematurely. And that would be a shame, I'm sure you agree.

You should devote some time to a ritual that will protect you. Like a waltz, it has three steps.

1. **Moisturize** Do it each and every day. There is no shortage of creams out there and all they need from you is one simple action: a gentle rub with the palm of the hand in a circular upward motion. Five minutes every day will be enough to stimulate the production of collagen, which will help the tissue resist stretching (collagen knows how to do this: that's its job).
2. **Exfoliate** Use a gentle product, with fine grains or no grains at all. The epidermis is at its most sensitive here.
3. **Protect** From what? The sun, of course. When it reappears in springtime, cleavages come out of hibernation. And ultraviolet rays hit the skin perpendicularly on this part of the body. So don't skimp on the sun-cream factor: a good 50 ought to do it.

Here are two more pieces of advice for **keeping your skin in good condition**:

1. Avoid extremely hot water coming into contact with the chest because it softens the cutaneous tissue. Better still: finish your shower with a jet of cold water. Yes, I know, it's a bit brutal, but your skin will thank you.

2. If you wear eau de toilette or perfume, give your clothes a spritz rather than your neck or upper chest. Alcohol dries out the epidermis and, having followed all my previous advice to the letter, it would be a pity to shoot yourself in the foot. Or the chest . . .

All clear? Good. That'll be all . . .

3

The fitness zone

Low-cost exercise

Now we come to the fitness zone. This chapter is principally aimed at people who do regular physical exercise or have decided to start. But everyone else is welcome too. You will find a few suggestions of ways to work your body without even realizing you're doing it. Or almost. I call it 'low-cost' exercise and it's about halting the catastrophic sequence that goes: the less we move, the less we want to move; the less we want to move, the less we're able to move; the less we're able to move, the less we move . . . Get the picture? This vicious circle of physical deconditioning is often responsible for inactivity.

It is self-perpetuating, dragging its victims to a place where their physique and overall quality of life deteriorate.

You can't make a leopard change his spots, so I shan't try and force you to do anything. But it is my job to inform you that you can carry out some basic fitness maintenance on your body while going about your daily activities. If you're doing these things anyway, you may as well make them serve some purpose. If you keep the following few suggestions in mind, you might move a bit more, which might make you *want* to move a bit more, and so on, until you're riding the vicious circle in reverse. Until, just maybe, you have turned it into a virtuous circle.

1. **Abdominals** Do you sometimes watch television? Don't say no, I won't believe you. So, yes you do. Carry on. But first, put a rug down in front of your giant screen. Lie on your back and pedal your legs in the air for a few seconds (or several minutes if you feel like it): this will build up your thigh muscles and your abdominals too. And you won't miss one second of your programme. I can't promise you a six-pack. But I can assure you that it will work off some of the wobble. A little bonus side effect: this exercise stimulates circulation and gives you an energy boost.

   Variation: lying or sitting, keep your legs outstretched in front of you and do a series of little upward lifts, raising your feet in the air. The only risk you run is of annoying the person you share the sofa with. But they love you; they'll understand.

   Variation on the variation: every 10 minutes, while sitting on your armchair or sofa, hold your legs out straight for several seconds. Now, this *will* help you get some abs back.

2. **Thighs** Are you ever on the phone? Silly question. While talking, stand against a wall and raise one leg up, ideally at 90 degrees to the body. Hold this position for a few moments, then lower the leg, and do the same with the other one. This exercise, if done properly, will help develop your thighs.

   Variation: knee lifts. Bend your leg at the knee and raise it as high as you can, keeping your torso upright. Hold the position for two seconds then return to the initial position without letting your foot touch the floor. Repeat the movement several times. Then start again with the other leg. And so on, until you feel the exercise is bearing fruit in the thigh and calf department.

3. **Calves** Cycling isn't the only way to develop the calf muscles. All you need is a chair. Sitting down, with your back supported and your toes in contact with the floor, raise your heels and hold them there for a few seconds. Relax, then repeat the exercise several times. This is a simple way to strengthen your calves. Do it at your own rhythm.

4. **Glutes** Find yourself standing up from time to time? I expect so. Pretend you're a principal ballet dancer: slowly lift yourself up on tiptoes, and lower. Lift and lower . . . This little exercise is easy to do when you're in a lift, the shower or waiting for a bus. It will do you the world of good.

   Variation: still upright, slowly lift your leg out to the side then return it to centre. Do several series, listening to your body. You will soon feel the benefits in your gluteal muscles. Don't forget to change legs: you don't want to be all wonky . . . You can also work your glutes in a coffee break. While sitting down, keeping your back nice and upright, clench and relax your glutes several times, without forcing.

5. **Arms** Now you have a bum of tungsten, get to work on your arms. When you have a spare moment, simply stand up, making yourself tall, and stretch your arms out to the side, one at a time. Easy? Come back and say that after 50 reps . . . This exercise uses the weight of your body to develop your muscles.

As you can see, daily life offers hundreds of opportunities to work your body without cluttering the place up with equipment or impinging on your time. The smallest of efforts is never in vain: it all counts.

The magic of endorphins

They are called happiness molecules, and they have the potential to make us euphoric, mirroring the effects of morphine, whose name they partially share; they are, of course, endorphins.

The brain releases endorphins when we exercise. To be precise, the hypothalamus and the pituitary gland secrete them, providing you with the most natural drug available. Of course, you have to do your bit: you don't get something for nothing. You might want to choose one of the more 'endorphic' forms of exercise. There is an infinite variety: cycling, swimming, cross-country skiing, snowshoeing, rowing, step classes and, last but not least, jogging, the king of fitness. In fact, endorphins are sometimes known as the runner's drug.

Many elite athletes have spoken about what they call 'runner's high'. Thankfully, amateurs get a look-in too. They also recognize the moment, sometimes after a tough start to training and thoughts of 'What on earth am I doing?', when they sense they are gradually reaching an exhilarated state that makes them feel mentally strong. Of course, this is earned pleasure, endorphin levels being directly linked to the amount of exercise you do. You can't just gambol about for 10 minutes and hope to feel the rewards. The process is set in motion by sustained effort: the equivalent of half an hour of running at what endurance athletes call a comfortable pace (between 50 and 70 per cent of heart rate reserve). This causes the release of five times more endorphins than when the heart is in a resting state. And the sensation of well-being outlasts the period of exercise.

Endorphins' magic powers don't stop there. They are said to have an anxiety-reducing effect. Or so says a researcher from France's Institute of Aerospace Medicine, whose studies have led him to conclude that people who exercise regularly are less prone to stress than people who don't exercise.

Endorphins act as a pain barrier too. They work by attaching themselves to specific receptors that subsequently block the transmission of pain signals. As a result, the sensation of pain is reduced or even disappears. Now, don't go thinking that if you sprain something while out running you won't feel a thing because you're busy secreting endorphins. The point is, endorphins alleviate pain associated with performance. They soak up the effort. Just ask a top rugby player. Have you seen what they go through during a match? But they pick themselves back up. The players don't really feel the effects of the knocks and falls.

Endorphins also protect you from tiredness, up to a point. They act like a regulator that limits shortness of breath and muscular fatigue. Endorphins' last magic power: they play a role in sugar regulation during exercise. They limit immediate sugar consumption (fat is left to take up the slack) and this enables the body to hold out longer.

There you have it, the magic of endorphins in a nutshell. They're at your disposal. They're free, they're a gift, they're for you, they're *in* you. Just help yourself. Get moving!

Getting back into exercise: slowly but surely

You want to take up exercise again? Wise decision. And congratulations: it is probably the best idea to pop up between your ears since something foolish possessed you to stop in the first place. You will soon feel the benefits of this decision, physically and mentally.

Your first aim should be to avoid injury, given your body has got out of the habit of bending and stretching. So, whatever exercise you choose, always remember to warm up. A few minutes of jogging will suffice. You can even do it on the spot. The important thing is for your heart to receive the signal that you will be needing it to oxygenate muscle tissue. Then give yourself a kick up the arse (literally) by flicking your ankles up to your bum. The temperature of your leg muscles will rise, reducing the risk of a tear.

Obviously, the rustier your body, the more reminders it needs about moving around safely. You'll need to work on your balance. How? Easy! Pretend you're a flamingo. Just stand on one leg for about 30 seconds while doing a few movements with your body:

- Standing on your right leg only, lower yourself by bending at the knee.
- Rotate your chest to the right.
- Then rotate your chest to the left.
- Stand up straight again.
- Repeat the process balancing on your left leg.
- And again, right leg, left leg.

Doing this exercise about ten times will work the tendons in your legs and wake up the sensors in the inner ear. Yes, you'd never know it, but when you exercise even your inner ear has a job to do.

Two suggestions for people getting back into exercise:

1. Don't overestimate what you can do. Play to the crowd and you're likely to wind up in hospital.

2. Stretch at the end of the session. It only takes 10 minutes but it's vital if you don't want to wake up the next morning stiff as a board and aching all over, which is bound to make you feel disheartened and disinclined to have another go. And that would be a real shame.

Yes to exercise, but what time is best?

Exercise? Try and stop me. But when? In the mornings? Midday? The evenings? There is no cast-iron rule. But here are a few bendy ones for you; they will help you maximize the benefits physical activity has to offer.

A little fitness session of a morning is highly recommended, to wake up the body and its muscles. I advise cardio work, as long as you take it easy: don't forget you have got a busy day ahead. The main thing is to work up a sweat so you deserve that nice refreshing shower. The advantage of exercising in the morning is that you optimize productivity: endorphins secreted during the exercise session will help improve your concentration and creativity throughout the day.

At lunchtime, many people make the mistake of wolfing down some food then reaching for a pair of shorts, convinced that a bit of exercise will help their digestion. In fact, the opposite is true.

If you're moving, the body gives priority to the muscular work, and blood (which is needed for digestion) deserts the stomach and goes to supply your legs. As a consequence, digestion goes out of the window, you will be out of breath sooner and your energy levels will suffer. So, I advise lunchtime-fitness fans to take in provisions at around 10.30am, roughly two hours before their workout. Some fruit or cereal bars will do the trick. Remember to hydrate in readiness for the exertion ahead. Then, after the session, you can have a light meal, supplemented by a mid-afternoon snack.

Evening starts round about 7pm in my book. That's when your body is getting ready to sleep. Body temperature drops and so does blood pressure. Intense activity right now goes against these two natural phenomena. As a result, you might well have trouble getting off to sleep a few hours after exercising, and, if you manage it, a troubled night. So, if you're an evening person by nature, or because your schedule demands, it's important to choose relaxing exercise such as light jogging or stretching. Forget about breaking records towards the end of the day and remember this maxim of mine: 'Exercise at night, keep it slight!'

I repeat, although the morning is preferable, there are no rules. It's important to bear in mind that people have their own natural rhythms. Mind you, that leads me to a controversial question, and one that could easily throw my previous comments out of the window: do rhythms create habits or habits create rhythms? I'm convinced we can impose new rhythms on our bodies. So, I say to evening people, or those who *think* they are evening people (sometimes we pay too much attention to ourselves), try the morning instead. Just to see. You might be converted.

The unavoidable winter jogs

It's a funny thing: when winter comes around going out for a run seems less appealing. But it's got to be done. Don't give in. Motivate yourself. Have no fear of the rain and the cold. I've got a few tricks up my sleeve. I've tested them and they work. Have a go and see for yourself:

1. **Warm up indoors** Raising the body temperature and getting the muscles warm will improve your joints' flexibility. Your movements will be better coordinated.
2. **Think insulation** Your motto should be 'three layers': the first for breathability, the second for insulation, the third for protection. If it's really freezing you can wear the famous 'second skin'. Light, soft and engineered for the job, this base layer will enable you to retain your body's heat without hindering movement.
3. **Wear dark clothes** Murky colours absorb the sun's rays. What do you mean there isn't any sun? Of course there is. Otherwise it would be night-time!
4. **Protect the body's extremities** Find a hat, neck-warmer, gloves and socks for your head, neck, hands and feet. And choose materials with thermal insulating properties.
5. **Hydrate** Just because it's cold doesn't mean you won't get thirsty. On the contrary, breathing cold air speeds up dehydration.
6. **Keep yourself going** A few pieces of fruit or cereal bars will provide you with the sugars you need: your muscles need some to combat the cold and give you energy.
7. **Use your nose *and* mouth** If your workout isn't too intense, you're better off breathing in through your nose and out through your mouth. The cold air will be slightly warmed before it arrives in your lungs.

These tips will help you get the best out of your exercise session but it will be ruined if you don't have suitable footwear. Choose a pair of trainers that will keep your feet dry. Some have a waterproof membrane on the inside to protect you from the rain.

Water post-exercise: fizzy or still?

Once you've finished your exercise session it is essential to rehydrate. And now you have a major dilemma. Still water or sparkling water? With or without bubbles? There are certainly more pressing questions. But it's worth knowing that your choice depends on the nature of the activity.

At the end of a gentle yoga, dance or keep-fit class, you can rehydrate with still water. If, on the other hand, you've treated yourself to a workout of more than three quarters of an hour, if you have demanded a lot of your body, as you might during a bike ride, a run or several lengths in the pool, if you have worked up a sweat basically, go for sparkling water. It is generally richer in salt, which is appropriate for the body when it has lost sodium through physical effort.

Of course, it all comes down to taste. Although it doesn't contain calories, sparkling water has a particular flavour. The bubbles prickle the mouth slightly. It almost feels like swallowing something. As a consequence, it accentuates the sensation of 'feeling full', which is worth knowing if you're someone who wants to eat less.

But there are downsides to fizzy water. Drinking it means you are swallowing gas. Gas that, sooner or later, must be expelled. And if, by any chance, you have a fragile stomach and a few little gastric issues, even short-lived, well . . . I'm not going to draw you a picture.

To sum up: sparkling or still, the choice is yours; the most important thing to remember is always hydrate and always rehydrate.

What about **tap water**? It doesn't always have a good reputation and that's a pity because it is good. For people who exercise and everyone else. Squeezed by marketing gurus on one side and insistent-looking waiters on the other, we consumers sometimes feel duty bound to consume bottled water. And we pay the price. A price up to 300 times higher than tap water, which in France costs around 0.35 centimes a litre. Bear this in mind: even though the taste can vary from one town to the next, or even one neighbourhood to the next, tap water will never do you any harm. It is a healthy product, probably regulated more stringently than any other food and drink on the planet.

Pull your socks up

Here's a question for those of you who have a sporty lifestyle and don't baulk at a bit of physical effort: have you heard of recovery socks? Now, hang on: I'm not talking about some old pair you find in the back of a drawer. 'Recovery socks' are also called compression stockings. They can help you recover from physical effort.

A passing fad? Far from it.

When you exercise, your body's cells produce waste that tends to stay in the lower, weight-bearing parts of the body (unless you can run a marathon standing on your head . . .). If toxins pool in the muscles you are bound to get 'heavy legs'; muscular recovery becomes more difficult. You need to facilitate the draining process.

How? By improving what we call venous return.

Recovery socks (or compression stockings) exert pressure around the veins of the leg, preventing blood and waste matter lingering in the lower limbs. They work a bit like a pump: with each muscle contraction the blood is gradually squeezed up the leg, bringing it closer to the organs that will filter it.

Ideally, go for socks that cover the whole leg, from the feet to the thighs. But not all forms of exercise lend themselves to such an outfit . . . The main thing is that they cover the ankles and calves, where blood is most likely to pool.

Cramp: when muscles get carried away

If you enjoy exercising, you will know about cramp. You may even have suffered from it. Yes, I know it hurts . . . It's handy to know how to avoid it and how to treat it when it does occur.

Cramp is to an athlete what a power cut is to someone who works in IT, or a rail-workers' strike is to train travel: everything stops. The reason for it is simple: one or more of your muscles has contracted involuntarily.

Of course, you're more prone to cramp when you exercise because you're asking your muscles to work. They fill up with waste matter and toxins that reduce their output and capacity to tolerate effort. If you pull too hard on a piece of string there is a danger it will break.

So what should you do when the pain strikes?

One thing and one thing only: massage it. But you have to massage in the opposite direction to the contraction; the idea is to stretch the muscle. Let's take the calf muscle as an example. It contracts. Instead of screeching, rub, having first flexed your foot, i.e. point your toes up towards you.

Of course, the best way to fight the pain is to make sure cramp doesn't strike in the first place. Because it never comes on by chance.

It is vital you start your workout with a few minutes' warm-up and remember to hydrate before, during and after exercising. It's just as important to use the proper equipment and listen carefully to any technical instructions you may be given. A false movement or an incorrect pose can bring on cramp.

Clever Dicks say that the best way to avoid cramp is not bothering to do any exercise in the first place. Not wrong. But not entirely right either. Your body needs a minimum amount of physical activity. I encourage you to move more. Regular training will help your body get used to working out and, in time, it will get used to preventing cramp too.

Exercise and bras

With your permission, all you active women, I would now like to turn my attention to your breasts. You have to look after them and most of you fail to do so by not wearing a suitable bra when you exercise. But, I hear you say, what is a suitable bra?

A suitable sports bra is one that limits the movement of the breasts, which, without fail, will start to yo-yo when you move vigorously. Said bra will even help delay the natural sagging that occurs over time. Your breasts, which are basically made up of glands and fat tissue, are held together by very fine ligaments. During exercise, they are subjected to movements of varying intensity which can cause these ligaments to tear. Long term, this is bound to cause sagging. And once your breasts are no longer supported by these ligaments, there isn't much you can do about it. No toning exercise, no non-surgical solution, in fact, can return them to their initial firmness. Now, I'm not saying for a moment that there is no point doing specific exercises (on the whole, they tend to work the pectorals): they can be very effective indeed, but only if you do them *before* maximum droopage has set in.

I'm not going to start praising this or that brand of bra, but I think you should go for a very rigid one without underwiring. Ideally, you should have several, because wearing them too often can make them go soft (the bras, not the breasts).

Some of you will complain that Mother Nature did you a disservice, believing women with small breasts can get away without wearing a bra to exercise. Not so. All breasts, even small ones, move. Certain scientists, some of them men with a knack for combining business and pleasure, have gone so far as performing tests and their conclusions are irrefutable: for A and B cups, the amplitude of movement can reach 4cm in relation to the resting position. Of course, that's a long way from the 14cm recorded for more ample breasts, but still.

So, I say again, don't discount the sports bra, available in specialist shops. It will reduce breast movement by 75 per cent, compared with 40 per cent for a regular bra. If required, do add pads and perhaps apply grease to the nipples to avoid any irritation.

Exercise and periods

If you're a woman who enjoys exercising, you might sometimes feel a bit under par when the planned fitness session coincides with your period. This is only to be expected: the drop in energy is due to a slight loss of iron. And iron is important: it is transported to the muscles where it helps oxygen attach itself to red blood cells. See the pattern? Less oxygen, less energy, less performance, less puff, less desire to get moving in the first place.

In these circumstances I wouldn't blame you for skipping a workout or two. But you can also sidestep the problem by compensating for the absence of iron. During your period, it's a good idea to fill up on beans, lentils, chickpeas and soya (any legumes basically). These will work wonders, as will red meat, shellfish and fish. Add a few nuts too, such as almonds or hazelnuts, and you'll never go short. In fact, when it comes to exercise you'll be iron-willed!

Exercise and pregnancy

Exercising when pregnant? Yes, of course! I won't go as far as recommending you imitate Laurence de la Ferrière who, a few years ago, recounted her adventures at 8000 metres while five months pregnant (an exploit that required several months of acclimatization and could only be attempted by a top athlete), but I do strongly advise you to exercise, provided your pregnancy is progressing normally, you gradually reduce intensity as the weeks go by and, it goes without saying, your doctor hasn't prohibited it.

It is important to take some precautions:

1. No working out in hot and humid conditions.
2. No high-altitude activities, beyond 2500 metres.
3. No underwater diving, owing to the change in pressure and the fact we don't yet fully understand what effect the bottles' mix of respiratory gases has on the foetus.
4. Your exercise session must not make you exceed a body temperature of 40 degrees. Don't worry, you won't have to lug a thermometer around: such temperatures are only reached during extremely intense effort.

Apart from that, you have the all-clear, or almost . . . Be aware that the specialists (and I defer to them) have got together and agreed that a pregnant woman's pulse rate must not exceed 70 per cent of her theoretical maximum. Calculating this is disconcertingly simple: start with 220, subtract the future mother's age and work out 70 per cent of that.

Still confused? Get out your calculators. I'll use a 35-year-old mum as an example. Please show your working:

$$220 - 35 = 185$$
$$185 \times 0.7 = 130$$

Conclusion: our mum of 35 must not exceed 130 heartbeats per minute while working out. That's handy, as it roughly corresponds to a sustained brisk walk. Walking is a form of exercise I recommend for pregnant women, along with swimming. The latter cuts out impact, which means you avoid joint trauma, and you also benefit from water's natural massaging effect, which is good for you and good for your baby.

The advantage of exercise during pregnancy is that it prepares you physically for a very physical event. Giving birth is hardly run-of-the-mill. You ought to allow two months after the birth of your child before returning to exercise proper (four in the case of a Caesarean). After that? Some would say bringing up a child is a sport in its own right . . .

Aqua biking: pedalling underwater is all the rage

Aqua cycling, hydro-spinning, pool biking . . . Call it what you want, just get used to the idea: this form of exercise is getting more and more popular.

How does it work? It's stunningly simple: you sit on an exercise bike as normal, except you're in your swimsuit . . . And the bike is in a swimming pool . . . And the pool is full of water . . . And that changes everything.

In the pool, your heart beats less quickly than in the open air, which means you're likely to impress yourself. Because it's submerged, your body is lighter. So you feel less effort even though your muscles are working hard to push against the weight of the water. Classes tend to last no more than an hour and you will have burnt more fat than you might think before you've even had a chance to complain about feeling tired!

And the benefits of aqua biking don't stop there. This activity rapidly develops your lower body, from calves to back via thighs, glutes and abs. And there is no impact, so it saves your joints. Just imagine: the water actually strokes you as if you were a cat. This is the only form of exercise I know of where a massage is provided *while* you work out. A perpetual massage, due to the motion of the water. Nice, eh?

This fashionable pursuit could be a good opportunity for people who usually shun exercise to take the plunge. Mind you, you might have to splash the cash too. Aqua biking isn't always cheap. People who are lucky enough to have access to a municipal pool with group lessons partially funded by their local authority should make the most of it.

There is an alternative if you live by the seaside: *la longe-côte* (literally 'follow-coasting'). In France, this form of exercise is attracting more and more participants of all ages. It's good for your back, your heart and your balance, it doesn't harm your joints and you're free to vary the intensity of your workout. It involves walking or running chest-deep in the sea, following the coastline, as the name suggests. You can do it in groups and chat as you go. People do it in spring, summer, autumn and winter too, provided they are equipped with a neo-prene suit.

Nordic walking

Now, concentrate: *sauvakävely*. Sound familiar? No? Thought not. Unless you happen to have a degree in Finnish. *Sauvakävely* isn't the name of a volcano; it's the Finnish for Nordic walking. This form of exercise, which is rapidly gaining in popularity, comes to us from Finland.

Basically, Nordic walking is cross-country skiing without the skis, without the snow, without the weekly ski pass and without *tartiflette* at €50 the slice. All that really leaves is the poles. But that's actually quite a lot. Nordic walking is a complete joy to learn, very nearly as fun as pétanque, I'd say . . . Hard to think of anything simpler: while walking, you accentuate the natural movement of the arms and propel yourself forwards with the help of the two sticks.

This activity has hundreds of benefits. You can do it at any age, whatever condition you're in, by yourself or in a group. It's ideal for people who don't call themselves sporty but could be tempted into doing a bit of exercise. The movement requires your muscles to work in harmony: arms, pectorals, shoulders and bum. The body is invigorated, you breathe better and, as a bonus, you get to enjoy some beautiful scenery.

To sum up, much like the Lottery, Nordic walking is an easy sell: it's simple, cheap and you can win big time. You just need to equip yourself with a pair of poles (a few dozen euros) to absorb vibrations on your behalf. Choose them carefully: multiply your height by 0.7 to work out the right length.

Body combat: fancy giving it a go?

Like fitness? Don't dislike martial arts? Or vice versa? Here's a form of exercise that you probably haven't considered: body combat.

I won't claim it's the latest thing because the concept has been around for fifteen years or so. It is the brainchild of a New Zealander who thought it would be a way to let off steam and have fun while giving the body a total workout.

Classes generally last an hour. You 'fight' yourself, but you do so with other people and to music that has been especially chosen for the purpose: it's usually dance music with rhythms designed to accompany your cardiac activity. Body combat really gets your heart rate up. It also improves your stamina and muscle development. The thigh muscles have got their work cut out (you will find yourself jumping and high-kicking an invisible adversary, maintaining your balance as best you can), and the shoulder and arm muscles are busy too (you do combinations of uppercuts, left hooks and the like).

At this level of intensity, you're sure to offload stress and burn between 700 and 800 calories (over a one-hour session without much let-up).

Playful rather than violent, invigorating rather than dangerous, body combat is flourishing. And continuously evolving too, because every three months the routines change.

How about stepping into the ring?

Combat sport? It's not really the first thing that comes to mind when we decide to take up exercise. But it needn't be all about whacks and smacks and biffs on the nose: there are plenty of other possibilities out there.

Boxing? Welcome to the ring. We're talking about a gentler version of boxing here, not the traditional variety where sooner or later you end up having your face sewn back together. That's not the aim of the game at all. This is **kickboxing**, a discipline that combines kicking and punching, but a light-contact version: you're aiming to glance your opponent rather than knock them out.

Still turned off by boxing? And after I put the case so delicately? Why not try **judo**? Welcome to the tatami. This is the ultimate defensive sport: you exploit your opponent's strength to throw them to the floor, and occasionally pin them there. Judo is a form of ju-jitsu, a martial art combining combat techniques that originated in feudal Japan. It strengthens control of mind over body. And without putting yourself in harm's way because (would you believe?) ju-jitsu means 'the gentle art' in Japanese, a language I speak fluently, obviously.

No? Not judo? What about **fencing**? Welcome to the piste. Now, here's a sport that develops concentration and channels stress. Épée, sabre or foil in hand, you can take it up at any age. It's excellent for your waistline, strengthens the heart, sculpts you one hell of a figure and shy people love it because they get to hide behind a mask.

Not that either? You won't 'engage'? (That's how they say it in the glamorous world of fencing . . .)

I know. Let's try **karate**. Welcome to the world of dodge and block. This sport is built on these principles and is excellent for people who are more suited to evading blows than dishing out big hits. Karate builds stamina, flexibility, tone and speed.

Whichever of these sports you choose, rest assured that although they sometimes still have violent associations, today you can practise them entirely safely. And the physical benefits they offer double as psychological ones: yes, you will work your bodies in a ring, on a tatami or a piste, but you will also improve your self-knowledge and gain confidence too. And self-confidence is the name of the game.

Breathe and move

For those of you who don't see yourselves on a tatami or in a ring, there are gentler ways of keeping fit.

Stretch classes, for example, improve flexibility. A frightening prospect because you're stiff as a board? My point exactly . . . But if you work with your breath as you stretch, you will find you're suppler than you thought.

Some of the positions you adopt in a stretch class come from **yoga,** another gentle form of exercise from far away, both geographically and temporally since it started in India five millennia ago. Yoga is all about poses and breath. It increases our powers of concentration, helps reduce stress and strengthens our emotional control. And a distinctive feature of yoga is that it's open to everyone, including children, older people, pregnant women and people with disabilities.

Finally, from even farther off, you have **t'ai chi,** an ancestral Chinese martial art that has made a home for itself in the West. Unlike stretch and yoga, which are practised in all manner of positions, t'ai chi is always done standing up. This discipline values slowness and the movements are carried out extremely precisely. The challenging thing is to stay fluid and supple throughout. Mentally calming, t'ai chi primarily attracts older people who are anxious to improve their flexibility and strengthen their joints.

Stretch, yoga or t'ai chi. Take your pick. But go to a class if you can; first because it's more fun in a group, and secondly because you do need a teacher to show you the ropes and stop you doing a movement badly, which could have the opposite of the desired effect.

The mirage of testosterone

I'm not going to embark on another anti-doping diatribe – there have been so many – but I do want to dwell momentarily on a practice that can, I'm sorry to say, sometimes take hold in amateur sport. This isn't aimed at people who do a sensible amount of regular physical activity, but at the would-be champions who, having become fixated with beating their personal bests or the fact that their performance is declining with age, are prepared to deliver up their bodies and their health to some unscrupulous doctor or deal drugs in the back rooms of gyms. I would like to take a closer look at the psychological reasons behind the temptation they might feel (to alleviate guilty feelings) and warn them of the potential consequences (to prompt action).

Testosterone is the hormone of desire, of the libido, but also of muscles. Levels vary from one man to another: it goes from 2.5 to 10 nanograms (ng) per millilitre (ml) (a nanogram is 10 to the power of −9g). At 2.5ng, you have the strength and libido of a sea scallop. At 10, let's just say you're hyperactive . . . Doing intense exercise regularly (we're talking marathons) can cause testosterone to run low. Hence the temptation to dope: people look to rebalance their bodies by stuffing themselves with anabolic steroids in the form of pills, gels or injections. The desire to do this can become even stronger with age: from 50, a man's testosterone drops by 1 per cent every year. He also experiences such delightful things as muscle wastage, hair loss, strength reduction and fat retention, particularly around the waist. He may take it badly and the mean quips – jokes about bellies, baldness and 'no hard feelings' – don't exactly cheer him up . . .

I can't express this too strongly: do not get drawn into the doping mire. To begin with you need to know that anabolic steroids are defined as 'a drug that promotes tissue growth from nutritional substances'. In other words, it makes you gain muscle, which we've seen many times with athletes in the public eye. They go off the radar for months only to reappear more muscly than ever. Unfortunately, when they disappear a second time it's often due to the side effects, both physical and psychological. The list is long:

- tendon injuries: caused by too much muscle in relation to the tendons, which stay the same size
- acne

- development of breasts (in men)
- increased libido (great) and aggression (not great)
- growth problems and cessation of growth in children
- hair loss
- prostate and liver cancer (men)
- virilization (women)
- infertility or sterility caused by the reduction in spermatozoid production. The testicles produce sperm (their exocrine function) and testosterone (their endocrine function).

In addition to these disorders, which I should point out are mostly irreversible, suspicious changes may occur in the body. I recall those American athletes who all waited until they were 20 or 25 to be fitted with orthodontic braces. We were told this was part of a programme of body rebalancing, to improve their running technique. Taking anabolic steroids promotes some bone growth, notably around the lower jaw; some athletics stars find their lower jaws start to protrude and their teeth work loose. But please don't start thinking that a sportsman or woman who wears a brace is automatically suspicious. Good dental health, particularly for those who have made a career in sport, is a sure way to reduce muscle injuries.

An active person's to-do list

- **Look at the time** If you're leaping out of bed bright and early, remember your body is probably less awake than your mind. Before a morning workout, you must always plan to do a longer and more gradual warm-up than usual. Start with waking up the joints, carefully loosening your limbs, before moving on to the muscle warm-up and cardio work. The objective? To raise your body temperature. Sweating is a good sign: that means the warm-up has done its job, now you can go for it. Warming up is essential for all manner of reasons. You: 'Yeah, we know the rule . . .' Me: 'But it's always being broken!' A good warm-up, don't forget, improves performance, but it also reduces the risk of injury. It prepares you physically by raising your body temperature, and also prepares you mentally by improving your concentration.

– **Take care of your feet** There is a very good reason for this: a lot is asked of them during exercise. Physically active people must wear breathable shoes to reduce sweating and prevent blisters and rubbing. Shoes should also have good cushioning to minimize fatigue and relieve pressure on your bones, which can fracture. I don't want to alarm you, but stress fractures (fine cracks in a bone) occur far more frequently than you might imagine and, contrary to perceived wisdom, have a nasty habit of troubling people who are in great shape.

– **Learn to breathe** When you work out, it's important to get your breathing right, because the rhythm of your breath will influence your heart rate: if your respiration is all over the place, your physical capabilities will be affected. The first thing to do is to find your ideal breathing rhythm and match it to the rhythm of your movements. The best technique is to breathe out on the difficult phase of the movement and breathe in on the easier phase. And don't forget: to be able to breathe in fully, you first have to breathe out fully.

– **Use a heart rate monitor** That's not an order, just a tip. Visualizing the effort your heart is making during training can be very useful. The rhythm of your workout will vary depending on whether you're trying to lose weight or improve your stamina. Keeping an eye on your heart rate, and knowing your theoretical maximum, will improve the quality of your workouts.

– **Variety is the spice of life** Pecs, lats, abs . . . Do you feel like all your weights sessions are the same? Do you repeat the same sequence of exercises over and over again without knowing how to break the routine? How about shaking things up a bit? When developing muscle, it's good to vary your workouts because the body ends up adjusting to the routines you create and after a while it stops making progress. Every month, force yourself to change exercises or training methods. For example, consider circuit training, which strengthens the heart as well as muscles.

It's also a good idea for joggers to vary their workout: from time to time, try interval training, alternating between a fast and gentle pace. This method helps improve stamina and racing technique. Try a bit of sprinting, then a slow jog, listening to your body the whole time and never forcing it. And if, to start with, you have trouble keeping up this rhythm, just replace the slow jog with a walk. Interval training on an incline is a good way to develop strength and stamina at the same time. It's also good for building up the leg muscles and (you probably know this) the muscles of the upper body (back, trapezius, arms), which are made to work more when you are climbing.

– **Listen to yourself** When you're working out, you can sometimes feel unusual sensations. That's your body talking to you. So open your ears! Some feelings should alarm you: a chest pain, for example, possibly spreading down your left side, abnormal breathlessness or strong palpitations during or after your workout . . . These symptoms can all signal a heart problem. Stop immediately and call your doctor.

– **Take it one step at a time** France's former president François Mitterrand used to say: 'You have to give time to time.' Take a leaf out of his book. With exercise, as in politics, if you're in a rush you risk coming a cropper. That might mean an injury or simply a loss of motivation, which makes you feel like you're back to square one, physically and mentally. If, that is, you bother to go back to square one at all . . . All sports doctors will tell you: you have to gradually increase the duration and intensity of your exercise and, above all, never neglect the phases of your workout that seem annoying but are actually vital: the pre-workout warm-up and the post-workout stretch (more details below).

– **Stretch** Lots of physically active people decide they don't need to stretch any more. They either think they're flexible enough already or just forget about this fundamental phase. On top of its more obvious function of increasing flexibility, the act of stretching drains the muscles and this helps the body to recover better. It also promotes better blood return to the heart. Basically, dropping stretching can set you back. So make the most of the recuperation period after your workout: it will never be time wasted.

I'm aware that some people have recently questioned the efficacy of stretching, saying it is 'liable to lead to micro-traumas'. These voices should be heeded by anyone who has a tendency to push themselves to the limit. To them I say, stretching must never be painful. Everyone should proceed as they see fit, in an appropriate and measured way. In an ideal world you would have a massage as well, in order to increase muscle recovery. Now all you need to do is find a kind soul who knows how . . .

- **Pay attention to recovery** For a workout to be successful it's important to have recovered from the previous one. Because when it's over, it's not over . . . Recovery is an essential phase of any serious training programme. What are the rules to observe? Drink regularly, above all, and make time for regular and sufficient sleep. If you miss out on this phase of the workout you won't be up for the next one.

Fitness fans of the world, of all physical conditions and all levels, don't forget to stash an **ice pack** in your freezer. If you're suffering with a tear, a strain, a pulled muscle or bruising, you need to apply something cold to the affected area. As quickly as possible. If you're in pain you won't feel like dashing off goodness-knows-where to find something.

The cold helps reduce bruising. It slows down the influx of blood into the fibres. The pain is instantly anesthetized to some degree. That's why it's useful to have an ice pack always waiting patiently for you in the freezer. Just in case. Hopefully you'll never have call for it . . .

The things fitness fans should avoid

- **Drinking coffee just before exercising** A shot of black coffee might well be a French institution, but that doesn't stop it having a diuretic effect and accelerating the heart rate, which causes your blood pressure to change. Yes, coffee is a trap when it comes to exercise. It is supposed to wake you up and is known to stimulate brain function, so people assume it will make physical activity easier too. This is a monumental error. In fact, coffee reduces the flow of blood to the heart, which means the body is less well oxygenated after we drink it.

- **Exercising when there is a spike in air pollution** Even when the body is in a resting state, pollution has harmful effects on the respiratory system. So if you start moving it's bound to make matters worse. When you exercise, you speed up respiratory activity, inhaling outside air – and the fine particles that come with it – more quickly. Nasty things with poetic-sounding names such as ozone, nitrogen dioxide and sulphur interfere with respiratory mucus. They can cause coughing, shortness of breath and even chronic bronchitis.

- **Listening to yourself too much** If you're tired, you can continually put off the workout you've been planning. Stick with it. You will feel a lot better afterwards. When you're shattered, it's important to adapt the intensity of the workout and concentrate on the technical rather than the physical aspects. There will be time to set a new personal best when you're on form again.

- **Buying the wrong trainers** This particularly applies to joggers. Have you ever tried running barefoot? I know that some people recommend it but, frankly, it's pretty unpleasant, right? It certainly convinces you of the importance of having the right shoes. Running must not be taken lightly: it demands good equipment. Now, I know that shopping online is all the rage, but I advise you to take advantage of personal service in a shop when buying a pair of trainers. In a specialist shop you are sure to find a salesperson who knows their stuff and will treat your purchase seriously. If they offer to analyse your gait (by getting you to run on a treadmill) or inspect your old shoes to see how the soles have worn down, it's generally a good sign. If they ask you precise questions about the duration and number of kilometres you run, that's also a good sign. Do the trainers feel comfortable the minute you put them on? This is crucial and must guide your choice; don't worry about aesthetic considerations. A good pair of running shoes is a pair you instantly feel good in. End of story. I don't care if they're fluorescent pink or apple green. Also, be aware of a trainer's cushioning. It must be in the front *and* back. The front is important, naturally. But after a while, when fatigue sets in and you start to flag, the back is also important, since you hit the tarmac with the heel of the foot. Another recommendation: choose a size bigger than you would for your everyday shoes. That will prevent your toes rubbing against the end, because after a few kilometres of running your feet swell.

Let me say again, at the risk of repeating myself, that your shoes must be good quality, i.e. they must combine durability, flexibility and cushioning. Choosing the right pair will also stop you making one of the worst mistakes an amateur runner can make. Worried about their fragile joints, he or she deserts the tarmac and opts for footpaths instead, where the ground is softer. Bad idea. Yes, hard ground can be traumatic for your joints but it provides more stability. Good trainers are the answer.

- **Eating too close to exercise** Leave a gap of at least three hours between eating a full meal and exercise: that is the time it takes to digest your food. Elite sportsmen and women heed this advice, so there must be something in it, right? This leads us to another question: *what* should we eat before exercising. Have plenty of starch (pasta, rice, etc), lean proteins such as fish and white meat (chicken, turkey) and vegetables that are rich in fibre. But don't overdo it with the dairy products: they aren't brilliant for your tendons.

– **Hunger pangs** These are the enemy of exercise. And totally avoidable. Always carry something to hydrate you and something nourishing. And above all, don't wait to feel hungry or thirsty because by then it's too late. It's important to take the initiative if you want to guarantee the body is always fully fuelled. Drink regularly, a few sips at a time and, similarly, consider eating small amounts regularly during your run. Try high-energy foods such as cereal bars or dried fruit and nuts. Always have something on you.

– **Stopping for no reason** Giving up physical activity leads to a rapid drop in your blood vessels' suppleness. Eventually, the arteries stiffen. That's a shame, particularly since your body had got into good habits. Exercise has the distinctive feature of improving the capacity of arteries to alter their diameter, which enables better circulation and so better provision of oxygen and nutrients. This system helps detoxify the body by promoting the elimination of waste products and reducing their build-up in fat tissue. So if you're a fit person, my advice is: keep it that way.

Preventing osteoporosis through exercise

To keep your bones strong I suggest (you've guessed it) regular physical exercise. It's recommended as a preventive measure for osteoporosis, a skeletal weakness caused by loss of bone mass.

There are multiple risk factors for this condition: ethnic

origin, family medical history, excessive use of salt, coffee or tobacco, renal failure, inactivity, a deficiency in calcium, protein or vitamin D and, of course, age. Hence the pertinent question: does taking up physical exercise early in life have more impact on bone strength than taking it up later?

To answer it, 64 female tennis and squash players were selected and divided into two groups: those who had started playing at an early age and those who had started late. First observation: gains in bone density (measured in the humerus bone in the upper arm, the dominant one being the longer of the two) were seen in both groups. But the women who took up their sporting activity early had gained more. Conclusion number 1: to preserve bone strength it is advisable to do regular physical activity from an early age.

It is harder to evaluate whether the scale of the benefit varies depending on the type of exercise undertaken. One team of researchers did look into this, testing some 2000 men and women aged between 45 and 74, a time when they are starting to be susceptible to loss of bone mass, though at the time of the experiment none were showing any signs of osteoporosis or recent fractures.

Physical activities were organized into four categories according to their potential skeletal impact:

non-impact	swimming, golf or fishing
low impact	cycling, rowing or horse riding
moderate impact	martial arts, skiing or hiking
high impact	team sports, jogging, tennis or intense aerobics

The researchers then measured the bone density of their human guinea pigs. Conclusion number 2: the higher the impact, the stronger the bones.

But they also discovered something else: the relationship between increasing impact and strong bone density is accentuated by weekly activity for men but not for women. For them, a correlation can be observed for daily activity.

Overall conclusion: to build up and benefit from good bone strength, gentlemen should opt for weekly exercise, preferably high impact, and ladies for more frequent exercise, ideally daily.

4

How to stay in shape

Give your spirits a lift in 5 steps

Tired? Apathetic? Listless?

Just acknowledging this is a good thing; it's an invitation to do something about it. And the levers to pull in order to get your spirits back on an even keel are more accessible than you might imagine:

1. **Have fun** Ask yourself what you do for pleasure and what you do out of duty. Once things have been identified as one or the other, strive to put a bit more pleasure and a bit less duty in your everyday life.
2. **Avoid being alone** Make yourself spend some time with friends.
3. **Stay active** If exercise is a big turn-off, make do with some light movements or simply go for a walk. Whatever it takes to start secreting endorphins, the hormones that go hand in hand with your lust for life and your good mood.
4. **Go outside** If you are going to get moving, even just a bit, why not do it outside and make the most of the daylight? You should be on a permanent quest for sunlight because it loads you up with serotonin, which is an antidepressant.

5. **Think about what you eat** Go all out for foods that contain B vitamins, magnesium and zinc: they are very good for your mood.

Beat the post-holiday slump

We are prone to bouts of fatigue all year round. But there are moments when it's more likely to strike: a few weeks after the summer holidays, for example. The time off you enjoyed is already a distant memory and you feel the first signs of weariness setting in. It's virtually inevitable because going back to work means making an adjustment and surviving on less sleep. Plus, when autumn comes the days get shorter; the idea that the weather is getting worse subconsciously takes hold.

Are you going to just stand there, feeling helpless? No way! You've got to fight it.

The first thing to do is **prioritize exercise**. If being active is already part of your life, don't give in to a lack of motivation. If exercise is still an abstract notion to you, I recommend a bit of walking at least and, when the opportunity arises, taking stairs instead of the lift. It all counts.

You can **modify your diet**. Tiredness often indicates a shortage of iron. So, go for iron-rich foods: meat, fish and legumes, such as lentils or beans. Beetroot and carrots are in season in October.

You can also take steps to **enrich your leisure time**. Now is a good moment to get up to speed culturally. In autumn, a whole raft of new books are published and journalists are only too happy to tell us about them. Choose one: it will change your outlook and, more importantly, give you something to talk about with your friends and family.

Finally, there is something that will calm you down and get you back on your feet again: try **positive thinking**. Once autumn has arrived, it isn't too early to think about Christmas. What will you be doing? Who will you celebrate with? Someone needs to spoil your children, nieces, nephews or cousins. Ask them to start thinking about a wish list. Or write one for them. Get these things sorted now: it will lift your spirits, which is the first step towards getting in better physical shape. When the mind is heading in the right direction, the body follows . . .

The **flu virus** is back: it evolves quickly. That's why, if you are 65 or older, I advise you to have the flu jab every year. Don't let yourself be taken in by prevailing chatter that minimizes the danger of flu on the basis that most of the time it clears up of its own accord. It is an infectious respiratory infection that can lead to numerous complications and is sometimes fatal. It's as simple as that. Talk to your doctor: he or she will advise you.

Beat the winter blues

Winter, rain, snow, cold, gloominess and no desire to do anything. We all know the pattern. Feeling down? Chronically tired? Surges of anxiety? Chaotic concentration? Nothing going right? Take heart. Don't despair. It might just be a touch of the winter blues, a little seasonal affective disorder (SAD) that, as the name suggests, hits you in winter. It's not your fault in any way, and you can address it rather than just waiting for spring and the fine weather to return.

It's not your fault because the whole thing boils down to light. On a beautiful summer's day you get up to 100,000 lux full in the face (a 'lux' is a unit of brightness). It gives you a lift. In winter that can plummet to 2000 lux. That's low. Too low. And as a result you lose your mojo. Your biological clock doesn't work as well as it should. The secretion of melatonin (the sleep hormone) is light-dependent, so is inhibited during the day and stimulated at night. But on gloomy days, or when it's raining, the body secretes more, which leaves you feeling flat.

You can do something about it. Here's a radical proposal for you. Why not try a session of light therapy? Sunlamps often prove just as effective as antidepressants, minus the side effects. They are equipped with ultraviolet and infrared filters so your skin isn't at risk. You can hire one, you can buy one and you can even get one prescribed.

Relaxation is good for your back and everything else

There is a French expression for 'I'm exhausted' or 'I'm done in' that goes like this: *'J'en ai plein le dos'* (literally, 'I've got a full back's worth'). It's pretty apt: your body is in a state of tension and everything gets focused into the back. At times like this, a good route to explore is relaxation. We don't always think of it and we should, because it's something that is accessible to everybody.

Relaxation consists of relieving mental and physical pressure. It can be achieved with the help of exercises that make us mindful of our body and our thoughts. You can do it without specialist equipment, without signing up to the premium package at the local gym and without the need for an opponent. You just have to make an appointment with yourself: bring your body and a bit of time. You've got to admit that economically speaking it's a winner . . .

There are various techniques out there and they all aim for the same result: to free the body of tension. The environment must be favourable. You can't relax listening to 'Sympathy for the Devil' by the Stones playing at full blast. Make sure you have access to a calm room (semi-dark and a moderate temperature) and wear loose clothes, neither too warm nor too light.

Relaxation can be done:

- seated: try a comfortable armchair, with the back of the neck supported and arms lying on the armrests
- lying down: the head propped up slightly, a light blanket over the body, arms by your sides and feet apart

The idea is to empty your mind. To do this, you need to get rid of intruding thoughts and anything that can cause them. So, no smartphones within reach. Tablets are also banned; their blue light doesn't help you relax much (understatement alert). And don't even bother asking about the TV . . . The answer is no. Even on mute!

• Once your eyelids are closed, become aware of your breathing. Listen to it; savour the sound. Breathe in and out slowly and deeply. This calming rhythm encourages your body to relax.
• What should you think about? Your muscles. Tense them, then release. One at a time. Start with the feet, then work your way

up to the head. Take the time to focus on the muscles as you let them go.

- With your eyes closed, you are free to create your own perfect world. Visualize a colour. Your favourite. It could be blue, it could be pink. Visualize a place, an object or a situation that has made you feel good in the past. Fill your mind with positive images associated with happiness, success and a feeling of safety, whatever those things signify for you. Do you like the sound of the sea? Think of that. You like the smell of mint? Think of that too. Can you still hear the peals of laughter from that last get-together with friends? Prolong the pleasure: it's free!

I'll say it again: exercises like this are accessible to everyone. They seem banal and formulaic, but you can't begin to imagine the benefits they generate by reconnecting people to their inner life. My advice is this: relax in this way in the morning or after a day's work (before sitting down to eat). You can choose to devote an hour to relaxing or just spend 10 minutes, depending on your needs, wishes and the time available to you. Bear in mind that the more you practise, the easier it will be to reach a state of relaxation quickly. It's simply a matter of training. The body learns fast.

Prevent musculoskeletal disorders

Our muscles, tendons and nerves belong to the family that is referred to in physiological speak as 'soft tissue'. We need them to work permanently, which makes them susceptible to all sorts of pathologies: tendonitis (inflammation or degeneration of the tendon), carpal tunnel syndrome (compression of the median nerve in the wrist which causes pain in the hand and fingers, tenosynovitis (rheumatism of the shoulder, hand or foot), epicondylitis (the famous tennis elbow), hygroma (your elbow doubles in size, it's very attractive) . . . Never mind the fancy ones such as tendinopathy of the rotator cuff (you remember, surely: it causes pain in the left shoulder that moves over to the right one, or vice versa).

These conditions can affect nerves (a nerve becomes compressed and can no longer transmit the nerve impulse normally), muscles (a muscle contracts, the blood vessels tighten, the elimination of waste matter is disturbed . . . hello, lumbago) or spinal discs (making you a prime target for a slipped disc). All the items on this menu of delights are classed as MSDs (musculoskeletal disorders). They wreak havoc in developed countries, sometimes unbeknownst to sufferers because people tend not to pay enough attention to the early-warning signs. And yet they are easily identifiable. It is your responsibility to start asking questions if any of the following apply:

- You can't make the slightest physical effort without feeling aches and pains.
- You notice that you can no longer do physical activities that weren't problematic before.
- You feel like ants have set up home in your hand (pins and needles, numbness).
- You notice continued and unexplained loss of sensation.
- You have chronic stiffness and frequent cramp.
- One of your fingers keeps giving you the finger, i.e. bends without you telling it to.

Stress, excessive effort, sedentary work and repetitive movements can all cause symptoms to appear. They are more likely to strike in winter as the cold tends to makes matters worse.

But there is a way to limit the damage: don't get these disorders in the first place. To help honour this statement of the obvious, I would like to introduce you to certain preventive measures:

Beat neck pain

– When was the last time you changed your pillow, I wonder? That is not an idle question: a healthy neck goes to bed on a good-quality pillow, i.e. not one that is worn out. It's important to choose a pillow that corresponds to your sleep habits.

  If you snooze on your side, your pillow should be thick, to keep your neck cervical vertebrae in good order. You prefer lying on your back? No problem: buy yourself quite a firm pillow. Spreadeagled on your front is more your style? In that case, invest in a thin pillow that is flexible and not too bulky: it will keep your head aligned with your spine.

– When was your last eye test? And your last routine trip to the dentist? These are even less idle questions than the pillow one. Plenty of sore necks stem from dental or eye problems. When the eyes are tired the neck tenses, asking too much of the muscles at the base of the skull that, unfortunately for them, work directly with the eyes. And so the circle is complete. To break it, have check-ups once a year. And remember the simple things like an antiglare protector for a computer screen or adjusting the brightness (which you can alter throughout the day).

– Ladies, I know you keep your whole life in your handbag, so it's hardly surprisingly that it weighs a ton . . . Always wearing it on the same shoulder will end up making you unbalanced, a prelude to pain in the neck. Solution number 1: alternate between the right and left shoulder. Solution number 2: have a handbag clear-out to lighten the load. Solution number 3: carry around two bags (one on your shoulder and one in your hand), which will be lighter. Solution number 4: go for a rucksack, though it's not a great look when you're wearing a long backless dress.

– Smartphone and tablet addicts, may I remind you that it's important to keep the neck and back as straight as possible. Otherwise you're a prime candidate for 'text neck'. Make yourself position the screen at eye level, so as to avoid bowing your head or bending your neck. And if you think you can get out of it by telling me you always use the landline to call friends, it won't wash, I'm afraid, because I bet you wedge the phone between your ear and your shoulder. This movement, like all repetitive asymmetric movements, is banned.

– If, despite following all these recommendations, you feel neck pain coming on, tip your head forwards then backwards. Very slowly. Then turn it left and right. Relax your shoulders. And do the same again. I'll wager that will provide some relief.

Beat heavy legs

– Heavy legs betray poor circulation. You have to take action first thing in the morning when dealing with improving venous return (the flow of blood to the heart). It can be stimulated by exercises. Stand up straight, raise one knee and take it out to the side in order to open your pelvis, staying balanced on the other leg. Repeat this ten times on each side. Next, raise yourself on tiptoe then back on to your heels. Again, repeat ten times. This morning ritual wakes up the joints and muscles and improves circulation. It's nice and gentle.

- Jeans, stockings, socks, boots . . . If they're too tight they will affect circulation. Remember to loosen the vice from time to time by wearing baggier clothes and comfy shoes, particularly if you're taking a train or flying, when we tend to be cooped up in narrow seats. You can also try compression leggings, a comfortable alternative to compression stockings. Their distinctive material improves tissue drainage. No more legs like Babar the Elephant!

- In one respect heavy legs are like a dry throat: they should both have you reaching for a glass of water. Being well hydrated allows for good tissue drainage. Water leaves you cold? Try plant-based infusions such as red vine or horse chestnut: your herbalist will confirm their decongestant qualities.

- Crossing your legs while sitting in a chair can look elegant; it's also a good way to give yourself heavy legs, as blood tends to pool around the calves. The best thing is to keep both feet on the floor in parallel. Consider modifying the height of your chair to fit your body shape, so that your hips, knees and ankles all form right angles.

- A strong jet of cold water, starting at the feet and going up the thighs, will invigorate your legs. You can finish off the process by massaging your legs from the feet upwards with a chilled massage gel, straight from the fridge.

- From time to time, devote a few minutes to stretching. Sitting on the edge of a chair, extend your legs out in front of you. Tense them. Push your heels away from you (making sure they stay in contact with the floor) and flex your toes towards you. Hold it for 40 seconds.

Beat carpal tunnel syndrome

– We all have a median nerve. It comes down the arm and finishes in a delta pattern in the thumb and the index, middle and ring fingers. It can become compressed at the wrist, where it passes through the carpal tunnel; when that happens we feel stinging, numbness and pins and needles. Sometimes the causes are natural: hormonal or metabolic (pregnancy, menopause, diabetes . . .). But the syndrome can also appear after a trauma or, more often, because of the sort of repetitive movements familiar to DIY enthusiasts, gardeners or manual workers. People who are concerned should think about changing their grip regularly. They should also try to hold their tools with the whole hand and not just the fingers: this is vital to relieve the wrist.

– The computer has changed our lives. It has also brought about an explosion in the number of cases of carpal tunnel syndrome, to such an extent that it is one of the most prevalent work-related conditions in the developed world. You need to adopt good working practices and equip yourself accordingly.

Tool-wise, use an ergonomic mouse to avoid the line of the wrist being broken. Use a mouse pad with padded wrist support, which will relieve points of tension. Invest in an ergonomic keyboard: a two-part or narrow keyboard. With the first, the two sections are placed in line with each of your shoulders. With the second, you do away with the numeric keypad at the side, which means the mouse can be in line with your shoulder.

In terms of movements, try not to bend your wrist upwards: this action is terrible for the joint. Keep the forearm at right angles to the upper body and make sure that the point of contact with the desk is closer to your elbows than your wrists.

Beat tired eyes

- Your job might require you to read a ton of documents. To avoiding having eyes like a grouper fish caught in a deep-sea diver's torch beam, start by placing your reading matter 50–60cm from your face. By putting distance between you and the words, you're also putting some between you and tired eyes . . .

- Anyone who feels miffed about ploughing through pages and pages of literature, for work and not out of choice, should think about taking breaks. It's up to you how: go out for some fresh air for a few minutes, get your eyes working differently between pages by taking the time to look around you and into the distance, or maybe place a wet compress over your eyes. These will all provide some relief.

- The computer is often unavoidable at work. At home, on the other hand, you can decide to switch it off. This advice is basic common sense and I'm amazed how many people don't heed it.

Beat headaches

- If, despite following the above suggestions, you finish your day with a raging headache, I'm going to recommend something childishly simple: with your index fingers, massage your temples symmetrically and in circles. This will improve the flow of blood in this area. Often that's all it takes to give headaches the heave-ho. And it's cheaper than paracetamol.

- Headaches often betray neck tension. By stretching for a few minutes you will provide some relief. Here's how: tip your head slowly to the left, letting it fall gently towards your shoulder; do the same on the right side. Next, tip your head forwards, trying to touch your chest with your chin, then slowly backwards.

Repeating this exercise about ten times will reduce tension or even make it go away completely.

– Another remedy is water. Drink! Dehydration disturbs the flow of oxygen and blood in the brain. Which is why it can lead to headaches. From now on, start your day's work with a full bottle of water and tell yourself it must be empty by the time you leave the office. It doesn't count if you water the plants with it . . .

As you can see, pre-empting musculoskeletal disorders is a constant battle on all fronts. The eyes, the neck, the feet, the elbows, the wrists, the spine (and plenty more besides) are all interconnected. If one of them gets into difficulty the others will be affected. Have faith in a series of interlinked habits and practices, which must be adopted as soon as possible in order to avoid the scourge of RBPMSD ('really bloody painful musculoskeletal disorders').

Sleeping on the job

Sleeping at work? That sounds like a quick way to get fired. In fact, more and more companies don't mind their employees having a restorative nap. The practice was established a few years ago in Japan and it's been bearing fruit ever since.

Just to be clear, when I talk about a nap at work I don't mean a mega two-hour snooze, rather a moment of relaxation of 5–10 minutes. A trick for not ending up in the arms of Morpheus, and in your boss's office, is having a rest with a bunch of keys in your hand: if they drop (and the noise wakes you up) it means you were properly falling asleep and it's time to get back to work.

But since not all companies care about their employees getting enough sleep, and not all jobs are compatible with napping, here are some other ways to combat day-to-day tiredness:

1. **Make yourself take a break** every two hours, just like on the motorway. Often it only takes a few minutes, enough time to walk about, do a few stretches and get re-energized.
2. **Change activity** from time to time. If you've just done something intellectually demanding, switch to a manual task, and vice versa. You can always do some tidying up.
3. **Take the time to daydream.** Yes, daydream! Not for long: just five minutes spent thinking about something pleasurable in the past or to come. Sometimes that is all it takes to feel refreshed.

Along with the compulsory short walk during your lunch hour, these suggestions will help reduce stress and fatigue, both of which like to feed on your passivity.

Stretch the stress away

It is intangible, unfathomable and invisible but it can make your life a misery.

It likes to lurk in your muscles, which stiffen up as a consequence.

It is the root cause of a great deal of pain and discomfort.

I am referring to stress, of course. The most universal of modern maladies.

It's possible to fight everyday stress without turning your routine upside down or bringing your whole lifestyle into question.

How? By stretching. It's compulsory after exercise but short spells are recommended in the morning or evening too.

There are four sensitive areas you should concentrate on:

1. **The neck** This needs to be mobile and flexible. After all it's the junction between head and body. If it gets stiff, everything else will be affected. Often, taking the trouble to look after your neck will spare you persistent headaches.
2. **The shoulders** We all tend to hunch our shoulders and that promotes tension. By stretching this part of the body you encourage your ribcage to open and you breathe better.
3. **The back** *The* classic problem area, that comes up time and again in this book. Millions of people say they suffer from back pain. It's not surprising: we spend a lot of time sitting badly and we tend to slump. By being aware of this, you are already taking action.
4. **The legs** By stretching them we get the circulation going again, which invigorates them and makes them feel lighter. And when we're lighter we feel better.

Feng Shui for better sleep

Do you sometimes sleep badly? Yes? In order to improve the quality of your slumber, how about looking into feng shui, or 'wind water' to give it its literal meaning. It is a thousand-year-old art of Chinese origin and the objective is simple: to harmonize the environmental energy of a space in order to optimize the health and well-being of its occupants.

Of course, you don't have to believe in it. But it might be handy to take a look at something that seems more than a passing fad, to shake up our western habits. After all, a bit of curiosity never hurt anyone.

Take your bedroom . . . To arrange it according to the principles of feng shui, the first thing is to make sure your bed is well positioned. That means the head of the bed against the wall with space either side. So far we're pretty much all feng shui practitioners, right? Now it gets more innovative: the bed must not be placed in line with the doorway, as that could generate strong energies that impair the quality of your sleep.

A feng shui bedroom is free from anything that might emit electromagnetic waves: computer, television, mobile phones. But that's not all. Plants are sometimes too energizing so they're banned as well. It might be a good idea to diffuse calming essential oils instead (vervain, orange blossom).

Subdued lighting is also an important element of feng shui. So, don't skimp on the lampshades. You can even go as far as installing a dimmer. In general, anything calming is recommended. Some advice? Here goes. Walls? Pastel shades. Ceiling? Light. Furniture? Not too close to the bed because the energy needs to circulate. Pictures? Not brightly coloured ones. Mirror? Never facing the bed (risqué!) because it reflects energy. Bed itself? Wooden, if possible. Sheets? Cotton or linen.

It isn't my intention to make you move or replace your furnishings. I just want to make you aware that feng shui, which appeared in the West about thirty years ago, has gained more and more devotees, many of whom have rediscovered good-quality sleep.

Sleep apnoea: take action!

Are you among the 5 per cent of adults who are subject to sleep apnoea and endure its accompanying delights? You wake up tired, having disturbed those closest to you with unwelcome snoring, and things don't exactly improve over the course of the day, during which you are tormented by a terrible urge to fall asleep. This isn't a coincidence: if you've spent the night trying to get your breath back because you keep forgetting to breathe, it's bound to leave its mark.

So, what can be done to get back to restorative sleep?

Let's be honest: if you smoke, that doesn't really help matters. And then there's alcohol . . . The best thing would be to cut it out completely, particularly in the evenings. But I expect you're not averse to a little glass . . . You probably tell yourself it will help you relax and you'll sleep better because of it. Wrong! Alcohol is indeed a muscle relaxant but by encouraging the throat to relax, all it does is disturb the airflow. If you take sleeping pills they will have the same effect.

You can get dental devices that are designed to widen the airways during the night. These are orthoses. Unlike a prosthesis (which replaces something), an orthosis compensates for something. It is moulded to the shape of your mouth and brings forward the lower jaw and tongue. You won't look like George Clooney, I grant you, but it can be effective.

There are other treatments worth looking into such as radio-frequency (a technique for reducing tissue size), a type of spontaneous ventilation known as continuous positive airwave pressure (you have to wear a mask) and maybe even surgery. It's essential that you pick a treatment that is tailor-made for you. To this end, it might be useful to ask your GP for a referral to a sleep clinic, where they will know how to diagnose the problem and offer guidance.

Quell that jet lag

Everyone's had it, or will have it one day. Yes, you as well! It's hard to get around it, even though steps can be taken to limit the effects. There is nothing worse than treating yourself to a far-flung recuperative holiday only to lose the benefit as soon as you get home. You can just imagine the conversations:

'Whoa, you look like you need a holiday!'

'Thanks, I've just got back actually . . .'

The first question to ask yourself is what is the direction of your outbound travel: east or west? Shanghai or Los Angeles? Bangkok or Mexico? Because it's not the same. Before heading east, gradually shift your body clock by going to bed slightly earlier. Do the opposite for westward travel: go to bed slightly later. Do this progressively over several days.

During the journey, whatever your destination, avoid sleeping pills, limit your caffeine and alcohol consumption and, if possible, have meals that correspond to the time zone of your destination. And it's important, particularly if you happen to be a big eater, to eat lightly.

Finally, once you're there, adapt. If you're heading east, the trick is to make the most of morning light and go easy on evening light, and the other way around if you're heading west. In other words, be an early bird in Peking and a night owl in New York.

If and when you can get away, *bon voyage*!

Melatonin can help with jet lag but be warned, you should only take it if you are heading east, when your body clock is lagging behind local time. This will stop your body secreting melatonin too late. Consult your doctor first.

Flat tums and common misconceptions

How many times have I read articles that recommend ab workouts if you want a flat stomach? What nonsense! Anyone who thinks they can lose their spare tyre by developing their core is deluding themselves and has been sold a pup. When you do sit-ups you're working on your abdominal muscles. Very good. And where is the muscle? Under the fat! Should have thought of that . . . So the muscle is strengthened (which is a good thing) but the fat remains. And the only way to make the fat disappear is to lose it. How? It's back to the same old rules: adjust your diet and do some endurance training: long duration cardio work, such as running, cycling or swimming. It is thought we start to tap into the fat after about forty minutes of effort (jogging). That's when lipolysis starts; this clever-sounding Greek word describes the process whereby the body burns fat.

But it seems that not everyone is lucky enough (or brave enough) to experience this phenomenon. In terms of body fat, two out of six men are too round at 30; this rises to two out of three at 40. Things tend to get worse with age because muscle mass is shed over the years, giving way to fleshy tissue, which guzzles a lot less energy (and is a lot less aesthetically pleasing). The result: assuming constant activity levels, the body consumes

5 per cent fewer calories every 10 years. Factor in a less vigorous, more middle-class lifestyle (a taste for fancier food, for example) and you end up with a good layer of fat covering slack abdominal muscles.

Although it is never too late to change your lifestyle, I recommend adopting good habits as early as possible. On average, fat represents 15 per cent of body weight in a young person. Muscle predominates. And muscles devour calories. Making them work regularly helps them stay on message. The body has a memory, and it likes habits. So you have to give it some. And make sure they are good ones. Because it will happily sign up to constant dynamism *or* settle for stay-at-home comfort. The choice is yours . . .

Exercise after partying

The morning after . . . You're not on fine form and the mere thought of doing some exercise to blow away the cobwebs makes you want to die. After a night of dancing, drinking and possibly smoking, anyone who wants to stay in bed has a ready-made excuse.

Mistake.

What do athletes do at the end of a competition, when they're bound to be exhausted? Resign themselves to the inevitable recovery jog. The same goes for you: get moving, even if you're ready to drop.

Of course, I won't pretend a little nap isn't useful. 'Little' being the key word here. No question of spending the afternoon in bed. Doze for 45 minutes, an hour at the most. Next drink a large glass of water, and another one, then find the strength to give yourself a kick up the backside and go and do some exercise. Fatigue has you in its clutches? That is precisely why you need to swim, run or pedal. You're going to perspire, you're going to sweat buckets, in fact, and that's just brilliant because the perspiration will help eliminate everything that is making your head and stomach churn. The idea isn't to break any records here, rather to sweat out elements that are as undesirable as the substances the body produces when we work out. Goodbye, toxins. You'll notice that people who exercise regularly are better at handling the excesses of a big night than others, for the simple reason that their bodies are used to expelling waste.

After your workout, the comfort of a shower, or maybe even a relaxing bath, followed by a light meal will guarantee you a night of calm, deep sleep: just what you need to make you fighting fit again. The consequences of those revels will be no more than a distant bad memory.

The bike that rides itself (almost)

In France, around forty cities and towns offer self-service bikes for hire. In a few years, this bike-sharing scheme has become part of our lives. Anyone who has tried one will have noticed you need pretty good calf muscles to get anywhere. This innovation has given the bicycle a new lease of life. I'm sure it has also given a boost to another device that can accompany you on your day-to-day travels, whether that's a trip to the shops, going to work or even reacquainting yourself with the pleasures of a cycle ride without exhausting yourself: the electric bicycle. Why not give it a go? Sales are up and those who try it once don't look back.

An e-bike is fitted with a battery, usually hidden within the frame, under the pannier rack or in the chainset. You just remove it and recharge it on the mains.

There are two types of e-bikes: those with a motion sensor and those with a force senor. For the first type, motorized assistance is permanent: it kicks in after one complete revolution of the pedals. For the second, the amount of assistance depends on the effort provided by the rider. It's give and take.

What's stopping you test-riding both to see which one feels best? Nothing. Either way, it's 'small input, big output'. You're bound to fall in love with this gadget. As well as being practical, it might well bring you round to the idea of doing spells of exercise of whatever intensity you like.

There's just the small matter of the price tag. It can rise to several thousand euros but the basic model costs €400. If it gives you a taste for exercise it's worth considering.

Taking care of your heart

The heart, may I remind you, is a muscle. And like any muscle, it is strengthened by physical activity. This means we can re-educate it, train it and maintain it. That's why, throughout this book, I keep banging on about the need to do a minimum of exercise or, at the very least, walk every day. The reason it's so important is that as the muscle of the heart gets stronger, its nutrient blood vessels and coronary arteries become more developed, which makes it a lot more resilient.

Of course, few people can boast of living an exemplary life. Not even me, given my habit of eating charcuterie with butter. So, as time passes, you need to keep an eye on this essential organ. After

45, it's all about regular check-ups. Guidelines vary from country to country. (The following applies to France; why not go online to see what your government recommends.)

The frequency of screening depends on how many risk factors apply to you. Count them, from 1 to 10:

1. personal history of a vascular disease (heart attack or stroke)
2. family history of cardiovascular disease (at least one parent has early-onset heart failure, i.e. younger than 55)
3. family history of cardiovascular disease if both parents had heart failure
4. smoking
5. consuming more than two alcoholic drinks a day
6. being overweight or obese
7. having a sedentary lifestyle
8. hypertension (normal levels: < 140/90mmHg)
9. excessive cholesterol in the blood (normal levels: LDL cholesterol < 4.1mmol/L or triglycerides < 3.9mmol/L)
10. excessive sugar in the blood (normal blood sugar levels: < 6.1mmol/L)

If you don't have any of these risk factors, the following check-up every ten years will suffice: blood sugar levels on an empty stomach, abnormalities in lipids (cholesterol, triglycerides), full blood count, vitamin D3.

The check-up should be carried out every three years if you have one risk factor and every year if you have two risk factors or one major one (personal history of vascular disease or diabetes).

After the age of 55, it is important to have a cardiovascular check-up every 3 years: again, blood sugar levels on an empty stomach, abnormalities in lipids (cholesterol, triglycerides), full blood count, vitamin D3.

The check-up should take place every year if you have two risk factors or a personal history of vascular disease or diabetes.

The risk factors to consider are identical to those listed above.

The NEAT injustice

Are you familiar with NEAT? Chances are you're not. This acronym refers to the Non Exercise Activity Thermogenesis index, which relates to the energy burned by the body during involuntary physical activity. That includes various sorts of gesticulating, holding postures, spontaneous muscle contractions, basically all the movements that we do in a day without exercising in the strict sense of the word.

The NEAT index is a valuable way for us to unlock the secret of why some big eaters never get fat, and utterly infuriate people who only have to walk past a *boulangerie* to put on half a kilo.

Let me start by saying that the phenomenon of 'thin big eaters' is not specific to men. You'll find slim women who have second helpings of roast lamb. An experiment carried out by American researchers focused on 16 non-obese volunteers (12 men and 4 women), aged between 25 and 36. For eight weeks, they were made to 'overeat' by 1000 calories (a reminder: the daily calorie allowance can vary but it's normally considered to be 1800–2000 for a woman and 2100–2500 for a man). These human guinea pigs also kept to a programme of physical activities and an array of tests and examinations designed to evaluate energy output and body fat stored. The results? Each subject was ranked from

1 to 10 depending on the amount of fat they had built up. Some of them gained 360g, others 4.3kg! It begs the question, what had happened to the thin big eaters' missing kilos? That's exactly what the researchers wondered. And that's how the NEAT score was born, which enables us to measure the energy the body burns during involuntary physical activity. Some people are better off than others: it was found that the subject who generated the highest NEAT activity score burned energy equivalent to a brisk 15-minute walk every hour. Without leaving the house! Last clarification: women have lower NEAT scores than men. In other words, *Madame* burns fewer calories involuntarily than *Monsieur.*

That's just not fair, is it?

Well, life's not fair, as they say.

We are all unequal in the eyes of NEAT and there isn't a lot we can do about our score, which describes the energy we spontaneously burn just by being alive. Not a lot. Except, that is, exercise and keep an eye on our diet to ensure the body is functioning normally, i.e. the energy we burn is more than the calories we consume. Because, in the end, that's where the sensible solution lies. Energy consumption might well be higher or lower depending on the individual, but this definition of 'normal functioning' is universal. And the advantage of being physically active is that it enables us to consume energy constantly. By doing regular sustained exercise we also burn calories at night, do we not? This means the body is able to take in more calories than it otherwise could. This logic is exponential and works in the other direction too: the less we exercise, the more fat we produce.

So here's a neat way to get around your NEAT score: move more!

BMI: behind this acronym you'll find Body Mass Index, a notion conjured up by the Word Health Organization one fine day in 1997. This score can inform you of the nature of your body weight. It is calculated by dividing your mass (in kilograms) by the square of your height (in metres). Anyone allergic to maths who is on the brink of shutting the book, please don't.

Demonstration: I weigh 81kg and my height is 1.85m. My BMI calculation: $81/(1.85 \times 1.85) = 23.6$. I can deduce from this that I am a normal weight because my BMI falls between 18.5 and 25.

Calculate your own BMI and classify yourself accordingly:

BMI	weight category
less than 16.5	severely underweight
16.5–18.5	underweight
18.5–25	normal weight
25–30	overweight
30–35	moderately obese
35–40	severely obese
more than 40	very severely obese

Got your score? You know what you need to do . . .

Nicotine's *modus operandi*

I'll turn now to a matter that can be summed up like this: 'Don't smoke.' Two words say it all. If you already don't, feel free to go on your way. If, however, you're still lighting up, because of need, choice or lack of willpower, it means you haven't kicked a habit that is simply horrendous for your health. It's not possible to overstate this fact. Smoking is France's number one cause of avoidable death.

We can attribute 90 per cent of lung cancer cases and 73,000 premature deaths a year to it. It kills one adult in ten on the planet and is the second cause of death globally. Heart attacks, all types of cancer, strokes, acute respiratory diseases and more: the list of dangers that smokers are exposed to is a long one, although no one can claim immunity to health problems, of course.

Are you looking for an excuse? Here's one ready-made: your dependency is down to nicotine, a substance whose addictive powers the tobacco industry has done all it can to conceal. Nicotine goes in through the mouth, down the trachea, floods into the lungs via the bronchial tubes and enters the alveoli where gas exchange takes place. Crossing the walls of the alveoli, it enters the bloodstream. From here, it's on to the brain, which has nicotinic receptors. The nicotine activates and attaches itself to these receptors. That creates an electric signal and releases a chemical messenger (a neurotransmitter) called dopamine, which stimulates the reward centre in the brain. The dopamine released with each puff on a cigarette gives you a sensation of well-being: you feel liberated. The brain quickly adapts by producing more sites on the nicotinic receptors. When it doesn't receive its dose of nicotine, you experience withdrawal symptoms: addiction is established. You have to light another one. You're trapped. All the more so because nicotine burns calories. It raises blood sugar levels and so acts as a hunger suppressant, which is very popular with smokers who are watching their weight. It gives them the impression that cigarettes are an alternative to exercise and a good diet.

This purely physical addiction is compounded by a psychological dependency that is even more powerful. If this takes hold, you need to smoke a cigarette in order to think, relax and simply feel good. However, this psychological dependency only lasts a few minutes. We can make an effort to resist it. Give it a try. There is a wide range of possible tactics: drink a glass of water, have a piece of fruit, suck a sugar-free sweet, breathe deeply, change what you're doing or where you're doing it, make a phone call . . . The idea is to create a diversion, to dupe the brain and occupy the short period of time left vacant by the absence of a cigarette.

But kicking the habit is easier said than done, I realize. That's why nicotine substitutes have been invented. Via an inhaler or in patch, gum or tablet form, they provide you with a nicotine hit, removing the withdrawal symptoms. It certainly works and the advantage with these products is that they aren't toxic for the heart and lungs. They also do away with the smell of tobacco, which clings to interiors and clothes, and stop you suddenly becoming terrible company, two effects of nicotine withdrawal being irritability and aggression. If you've had your hit, albeit a substitute one, your friends and family can breathe a sigh of relief.

The genius of big business

The tobacco industry has been shamelessly lying to us for decades; we might write it off as barefaced cheek if people's lives weren't at stake. Who can forget that day in 1994, when the CEOs of seven tobacco companies affirmed under oath, before a commission of the American House of Representatives and with a solemnity worthy of the Hollywood greats, that nicotine was not an addictive substance? If you take an interest in advertising, have a quick search online: you will be stunned to discover the content of ads that would prompt immediate scandal if they were aired today. There is something for everyone!

In one, an seemingly authoritative man in the prime of life, proudly smoking, appears alongside the perfectly reasonable slogan: 'More Doctors smoke Camels than any other cigarette.' In another, we see a man exhaling his cigarette smoke in a woman's face: 'Blow in her face and she'll follow you anywhere,' says the slogan, presenting Tipalet cigarettes as an infallible instrument of seduction. This sort of nonsense made it possible to persuade many people that smoking was sexy in some way, whereas cigarettes actually impair sexual energy. An erection is due to an influx of blood and therefore requires a good blood supply. But smoking causes blood vessels to shrink. So blood flows less well . . . The cause? Nicotine, carbon monoxide, various free radicals and the countless other elements that go into a cigarette.

Of course, France didn't escape the steamroller of deceitful advertising. Take this third advert, featuring a couple. The man is sitting in an armchair, reading his newspaper while smoking his pipe. A woman (his wife?) is on her knees, looking up at him with a blend of adoration and admiration: 'I love it when you smoke your pipe and I adore Clan's unique smell,' she says to him (I gather Clan is a blend of pipe tobacco). I'm flabbergasted! Lying *and* misogyny, and in those days no one was remotely bothered by this.

It was another age, apparently a lucrative one for cigarette manufacturers. For a long time, a lack of organization on the part of consumers, people's credulity, the passivity of the authorities, the persuasive powers of the marketing experts and doubtless the silence of the medical world amounted to red-carpet treatment for the tobacco companies. For decades, they poisoned their fellow human beings without anyone batting an eyelid. Their imagination proved limitless. Once they had been unmasked, they were able to reinvent themselves, for example by introducing cigarettes that were 'flavoured' with menthol or fruits. Genius. A miracle of marketing. Believing they could spare themselves a few justifiable comments about their breath, it was mainly women and young people who let themselves be taken in, not suspecting that the freshness they felt with the first puff merely masked tobacco's often unpleasant and harsh taste. Not suspecting either that, insidiously, these innovations had made it even easier to become addicted, since the smoker tended to inhale more deeply.

Another huge con trick: so-called 'mild' cigarettes. Grasp this once and for all: a mild cigarette is still a cigarette. That's all that matters and it should set alarm bells ringing. 'Mild', so less dangerous, right? No, wrong, obviously. The composition of smoke from cigarettes calling themselves mild is virtually identical to regular cigarettes. The mild effect relies on the presence of little holes around the filter that dilute the smoke. And because it thinks of everything, the tobacco industry bombarded us with analysis carried out by 'smoking machines' that always draw on a cigarette in the same way. Except that a smoker with an addiction adapts how they smoke in order to absorb the amount of nicotine their body needs: they either smoke more or inhale more deeply.

All these acts of manipulation (this list is by no means exhaustive: I haven't mentioned roll-ups, for example, thought to be even more harmful than ordinary cigarettes) made the manufacturers a fortune and enabled them to sink colossal sums into publicity and marketing. Necessarily. The tobacco industry has always had its heart set on winning over new customers, only too aware its products kill half the people who use them.

It's never too late to stop

Some smokers think they are unable to live without tobacco, that this poison has become an integral part of their adult lives. They are wrong; they have miscalculated. It is never too late to get out of a bad habit, and this principle holds true for smoking. It is *never* too late. The number of times I have heard sexagenarians say: 'It's not worth it,' 'The damage is done' or 'You've got to die of something!' I would like them to take this fact on board: giving up smoking reduces mortality rates and incidence of disease, including in people who have clocked up thirty years as smokers. In the case of cardiovascular disease, the benefits of giving up are immediate. Yes, immediate! People quickly notice the beneficial impact on their quality of life. Live better and longer: doesn't that seem worthwhile to you?

Once you've made your decision, you need help. Do you have family? Friends? Now is the time to mobilize them. Tell them about the challenge you've set yourself and ask for their help. They will instinctively know how to take this news and how to pass on their respect and admiration. Never underestimate the importance of their role and the impact it will have on you. Just as the smoker's brain needs its rewards (provided in the form of nicotine), so the abstainer appreciates gratification (in the form of compliments, words of comfort and encouragement).

Give your campaign a bit of publicity. Inform your doctor, consider getting professional help and advice. If it helps, use social media such as Facebook, where you'll find friends, even virtual ones, who express very real goodwill. You're bound to come across people who have been through what you're going through; they will know how to offer support and you can benefit from their experience. Their enthusiasm and personal stories of how they got healthy again will motivate you. No one has ever regretted giving up smoking. On the contrary, people are proud to have pulled it off. It gives them huge self-confidence and enables them to achieve other feats they once thought beyond them.

The path is fraught with pitfalls, yes, but it's worth taking. Of course, you might crack. Don't panic if that happens. What's the point of stumbling if not to get up again stronger than before? The journey will have been all the more worthwhile. No one is immune to a relapse brought on by acute stress, a slump in motivation, weight gain or physical withdrawals. However, to fight against all that, you have a trump card up your sleeve: your ability to get moving.

Exercise (and this is hardly the scoop of the century: you'll read it time and time again in this very book) is good for you. And it's a great ally for anyone who wants to give up cigarettes. For starters, when you're exercising you're not smoking. That's one–nil to you against the infuriating need for tobacco. But, more seriously, you'll find that after a workout, particularly if you reach your maximum lung capacity, the desire for a cigarette falls away. Exercise is a tonic for body and mind. It increases the production of endorphins and so combats stress and depression. And since it is predominantly stress and a tendency to feel depressed that drive you to smoke (among other things), exercise helps drain cigarettes of their appeal.

Stopping overnight seems unrealistic? Tell yourself that others have done it. And if you need to go through a transition period, start by cutting down. This method works for cigarettes in the same way it does for alcohol: by having your first of the day later than usual, you reduce your overall consumption.

You have probably heard people say that the only way to significantly reduce risk is to quit smoking completely. Not wrong. For cancer risks, the fact you are exposed to tobacco at all is more significant than the number of cigarettes you smoke in a day. Even if you only smoke five cigarettes you are still taking a risk. But, again, smoking less can be a step towards stopping completely and it's sure to give you the opportunity to assess the benefits cutting down has on your health and appearance.

When you stop smoking, your complexion improves and the lines of your face become less pronounced. Tobacco harms the skin in two ways. First, the external effect of the smoke blurs the complexion. Secondly, smoking alters microcirculation, which leads to poor oxygenation of the cells of the dermis. Cigarettes also accentuate ageing of the skin by giving it a grey aspect. Stopping will definitely give you a brighter complexion. But that's not all: your powers of concentration will improve.

I often find myself battling the misconception that smoking helps you concentrate. The opposite is true: it affects memory. A smoker's brain cells (like the rest of the cells in their body) are less well oxygenated. Over time, that leads to an inevitable cognitive decline, which can be recovered a few years after quitting.

E-cigarettes

Since appearing on the market, e-cigarettes have sparked passionate debate. Some say they help smokers quit. For others, they are a hideous temptation: a so-called 'gateway' product. I am convinced that e-cigarettes are infinitely less harmful than tobacco. I wouldn't go as far as recommending that non-smokers take up vaping (we don't yet know the long-term effects), but I encourage people who aren't able to quit smoking tobacco to swap their regular fags for the electronic version: they will be shot of the poisonous tar and other carcinogenic products that tobacco has been shown to contain, and that is no bad thing at all.

Yes, periodically, studies come out swearing blind that e-cigarettes are harmful. Once you get past the eye-catching title and read them in detail, these reports are a tad opaque and prove nothing. Who finances these studies? It is often difficult to know. It's not hard to imagine that enemies of the e-cigarette might be trying to orchestrate a counter-attack. The first of these enemies is the tobacco lobby, for obvious reasons. The second, of course, is the pharmaceutical lobby: fewer smokers means fewer ill people; fewer ill people means fewer medicines, and fewer medicines means less profit. As for the e-cigarette's third adversary, people with a taste for scandal dare to suggest it is the state. Yes, the state! It's a bold claim, but their reasoning is worth considering. When a packet of cigarettes is sold, the state takes about 80 per cent in taxes of various kinds. That represents a honeypot of several billion euros in revenue, which would diminish spectacularly if all smokers took up vaping tomorrow, e-cigarettes being subject to far less tax. So, it turns out smoking is a good thing after all! But only for the public purse.

Exercise yourself off cigarettes

It's a rare smoker who doesn't want to quit. But one of the most common obstacles to giving up cigarettes is the prospect of gaining a few unwanted kilos. How aware people are of this obstacle is another matter. They say they're willing to make an effort but if the pay-off is a bigger bulge, it tends to make them feel discouraged. So they light another fag . . .

And yet, anyone who wants to get rid of this poison has an ally: exercise. You don't see someone put away a backhand passing shot with a ciggy hanging out of their mouth. Nor do you see joggers rooting around in their shorts for a lighter as they run past. It's an obvious thing to say, but when you exercise you don't do anything else at the same time. So cigarettes are out, at least for the duration of the workout.

Exercising also affects the desire to smoke. Numerous studies have demonstrated that moderate exercise for as little as 10 minutes has a rapid and measurable effect on the urge to smoke and on withdrawal symptoms. Any regular smoker who takes a modicum of exercise will tell you: afterwards it's nice to let the lungs breathe.

As for the fear of putting on a few kilos – as that was the issue I initially raised – exercise bypasses it. The more active a person is, the more control they have over their weight. That is blindingly obvious.

It's important for beginners with smoke-filled lungs to take things gradually. You can exercise with someone else or start on your own, alternating running and walking. This phase is vital: it lets you develop your base fitness. Then after a month those who want to can up the intensity and have a go at cycling, swimming, gym work or any other form of exercise.

Your progress will be a constant source of astonishment. Fat will give way to muscle. You'll find a tone and a muscular volume that will give you your figure back and increase your metabolism's energy consumption, even when resting. Keep up the training and you'll be caught in a virtuous circle, amazed at how much you're improving. And the explanation is straightforward: you have said 'no' to smoking and 'yes' to stronger muscles and healthier lungs. The quality of your sleep will also improve, which will lead to greater recovery, which will lead to better fitness, which will lead to an increased desire to get moving, which will lead to more progress. The circle is complete. Worth a try, isn't it?

Prevent constipation

Feeling bloated? Gassy? Appetite feeble? Stools hard and dry? I'll spare you any really gross descriptions. I mean sometimes I even . . . Okay, okay. Let's move on. But that's how it goes. I'm sorry, no one can boast of being completely immune to the symptoms of constipation. However, we can all prevent it by adopting a few good habits to keep things moving in the large intestine:

1. **Drink Water!** You had guessed as much, right? The tap variety is perfect. If you prefer bottled, choose one that is rich in sulphates and magnesium; it will help.
2. **Eat fibre** You knew that too, probably. You're more likely to find it in fruit and vegetables than charcuterie and pastries . . .
3. **Get moving** Physical activity plays a role in battling constipation. It is very effective, and the benefits will go way beyond your large intestine.
4. **Go to the loo** Well, yes! It sounds obvious but if someone is having a particularly busy day they can easily miss the window of opportunity . . . And that's unfortunate, because putting it off can make the urge disappear. As a result, the

stools dry out and their evacuation becomes trickier. It is important to listen to the body's needs . . .

Of course, if the symptoms are severe and your new habits have no effect, you need to see a doctor. Sometimes constipation is caused by something as simple as being on medication or having had a minor surgical procedure (the body has a memory).

Digestion? You're having a laugh

It would be foolhardy to ask you to laugh on demand for no reason. However, I must inform you of the benefits of laughter. They are numerous and one of the least known is this: would you believe that laughing aids digestion?

When someone laughs they contract their abdominal muscles, shift the position of their alimentary canal and get their diaphragm moving. We can't help it: it's a reflex. As a consequence, organs such as the stomach, the colon, the small intestine and the duodenum are given a massage, which improves their ability to digest your meal.

Consider too that laughing leads to increased production of saliva and digestive juices (vital to good digestion) and you'll start to appreciate that when you chuckle, a whole heap of things you never knew about occur in your body, and they do you good.

Now we just need to establish what gets you giggling. And what gets your friends giggling over dessert, say:

Have you heard the one about a bloke who's strolling through Amsterdam's red light district? He spots a girl in one of the windows and taps on the glass:

Tap tap . . . 'How much?'

'€400.'

'That's a bit steep!'

'Yeah, but it's double-glazed . . .'

You laughed? Happy digestion. You didn't laugh? Well, find another joke. But a funny one this time. And improve your digestion.

Gluten free is doubt-full

You find it in pasta, cakes, soups, sauces, bread (it's what makes it soft); we've always eaten it in the form of wheat and rye and now, suddenly, people start saying it's poison! There's a war on gluten. It's supposed to be infesting our food and responsible for all manner of ills: migraines, depression, nausea, insomnia, osteoarthritis, asthma, skin irritation, even multiple sclerosis and schizophrenia. I could go on.

A few years ago, the American cardiologist William Davis came out with a book in which he maintained that his patients were in fine fettle ever since giving up gluten. It has subsequently become fashionable. I've read that across the Atlantic one third of the population has tried to banish gluten from their diet (admittedly this figure is hard to verify, but the trend is undeniable), and I notice that in France we're heading that way too. Justifiable evolution or mass hysteria?

I'm mistrustful of fashions. They often mask juicy commercial operations. But I'm not deaf, and I have heard personal accounts from people who swear blind that adopting a gluten-free lifestyle has transformed their lives. The thing is, the doctor in me tends to rely on scientific evidence. And, to date, not a single study (I'll spare you all the contradictory details) has been able to conclude that gluten causes the ills listed above.

It's an either/or situation: either you're gluten intolerant or you're not. The first case has a name, coeliac disease, and is a recognized medical condition (1 per cent of the French population is affected). The symptoms are identifiable and the treatment involves a gluten-free diet for life. In the second case, and from a strictly medical point of view, the inclination to go gluten free comes down to fashion, auto-suggestion or cultural choice, and a perfectly respectable choice at that, I assure you. Albeit a restrictive one: it becomes harder to accept dinner invitations, buy food or go to a restaurant. It's true that businesses are getting organized: more dedicated food shops, websites and supermarket shelf space pop up every day. Needless to say, the products on offer are often more expensive than the regular versions.

A word about naturopathy

I belong to the medical fraternity. You find all sorts in our ranks, including nutritionists who tend to fall out with naturopaths on the subject of food groups. For some doctors, 'food combining' is bogus because it has no scientific basis. However, I can't bring myself to ignore the fact that more and more people are taking an interest in the naturopaths' approach, convinced they have better digestion when they obey the rules of food combining. They genuinely feel that to be the case. I respect this feeling and confess that it's difficult to come to a firm opinion, given that science is unable to explain everything. So, whether naturopathy piques your curiosity slightly or you think there may be something in it or you obey it to the letter, why don't I review it here, in a purely informative way?

For naturopaths there are good and bad food combinations just as there are good and bad clothing combinations. Put on a pair of red trousers, an orange jumper and a pink cap and you will immediately notice something's majorly wrong. Individually each item of clothing has its own appeal and usefulness. But put together they turn you into a parrot. (In his day the fashion designer Christian Lacroix dared match these types of colours to great cheers of approval, but not everyone is Christian Lacroix . . .) It's the same with food: apparently it's possible to make mistakes.

Take red meat. It contains iron that the body is very keen to absorb because it needs a lot of it. Problem: if you have a nice juicy steak with a tea or coffee, the absorption of iron is restricted. If, on the other hand, you add parsley to your steak, that's spot on, since parsley is rich in vitamin C, which facilitates the body's absorption of iron. Vitamin D, which we get from oily fish such as salmon or sardines, is an excellent companion for calcium (present in dairy products or spinach), whose absorption it promotes.

This means it's possible to believe you have healthy eating habits while still suffering from digestive problems, chronic fatigue or bloating, without really understanding why. If that applies to you, naturopaths will tell you the likely cause is incompatibility between different foods eaten as part of the same meal. Successful digestion is said to rely on the right food combinations. At the beginning of the last century, a certain Herbert Shelton advocated food combinations that were supposed to keep you healthy. A great many people still promote them today, even though they have no scientific basis. It seems it works well for them, and you can't argue with that.

To follow Shelton's principles you first need to classify foods into seven families. Some are larger than others and they aren't complete lists, but they all have their uses:

- Concentrated proteins: meat, poultry, fish, shellfish, eggs and hard cheeses such as comté, gouda, gruyère, mimolette or emmental
- Light proteins: almonds, hazelnuts, mushrooms, seaweed, tofu, soya and legumes (the most common being split peas, broad beans, lentils, butter beans or kidney beans)
- Fresh cheese proteins: yogurts, fromage frais, ricotta, mozzarella, cottage cheese, goats' or ewes' cheese, but always fresh
- Concentrated starches: rice, pasta, wheat, barley, rye, corn, wholemeal bread, etc
- Light starches: crispbread, bulgur wheat, cereal flakes, pumpkins, potatoes, chestnuts, etc
- Fruit
- Green vegetables, cooked or raw

Shelton advocates combining food groups that, together, facilitate digestion and absorption. To this end he suggests rules, including:

1. No concentrated proteins with concentrated starches
2. No concentrated starches with concentrated proteins and fruit
3. No fruit with concentrated proteins, light proteins, concentrated starches and light starches
4. Green vegetables and fresh cheese proteins go with everything

You have to say that's pretty restrictive. Perhaps a simpler approach can be adopted if we're suffering from weak digestion:

1. When you eat animal proteins, reduce or eliminate starch and replace it with vegetables.
2. When you eat starch, serve it with vegetable proteins or a small quantity of light animal protein (a boiled egg or a slice of ham). Vegetables are always recommended.
3. Try to eat fruit (particularly melon and watermelon) only between meals if you're experiencing bloating, and you notice that this makes a difference.

If following these principles makes you feel on better form, all to the good. Many naturopaths have come to believe that respecting these rules solves the majority of digestive problems. But we mustn't lose sight of the fact that things also depend on lifestyle, exposure to stress and a hundred and one other factors that make each one of us unique. Remember, whatever your objective (to keep your weight down, stay healthy, avoid digestive problems, for example) the most important thing is to eat modest amounts and take your time (chew, chew, chew). This approach will be as much help as all the food combining in the world.

Dare to have a cold shower

We spend roughly a third of our lives sleeping. It is essential for our health. But sleeping is not enough. You have to sleep well. It's crucial for sleep to be restorative if you want to avoid fatigue, reduced alertness, low spirits and mood swings.

One of the more original stress-busting solutions is having an early-evening cold shower, before eating. You're thinking the cold water will only wake you up, right? Wrong. The body actually needs a drop in temperature in readiness for the moment we slip under the duvet.

If you dare have a cold shower, go for 15 degrees. Once you've got used to it, you can always go down to 10 degrees, assuming you're feeling the benefits of this method. Take it gradually: hold the showerhead about 15cm from your feet before gradually bringing it up the body. You must always start from the feet. Relaxation is guaranteed: the cold will release endorphins (those well-being hormones) and chase away anxiety and stress that can interfere with sleep. And another advantage is that you'll learn to shower more speedily: you'll be in and out in two minutes.

I like/love/hate myself

You can't fail to have noticed that the concept of self-esteem comes up everywhere, particularly on the cover of magazines (especially women's) and in conversation. It boils down to the overall opinion you have of yourself, whether positive or negative.

Generally speaking, by the time we reach adulthood, the foundations of our self-esteem are in place, even if life's up and downs, be they professional, familial or romantic, can alter this perception. To a large extent, things are decided during childhood. Which is where parents come in . . .

The comments you make about your child's abilities can encourage or discourage them. It is vital that you have a good understanding of their strengths and weaknesses and that you help them become aware of what these are. And while it's important to give them ambition, you must make sure you don't pressurize them with unrealistic objectives. Not easy . . . Because if you set the bar in the wrong place – too high or too low – there will be consequences.

Low self-esteem inevitably leads to angst and complicates relationships with other people. It may cause permanent frustration, excessive self-blaming, constant undervaluation of oneself, impulsiveness and shyness, for example; and these behaviours can threaten the happiness of those who already have only residual levels of self-esteem. They might well stop them thriving personally or professionally. Troubles don't come singly either; it is common for low self-esteem to lead to depression, addictive behaviours (drugs or alcohol) or even a complicated relationship with food (bulimia or anorexia). At the other end of the scale, overly high self-esteem can lead to arrogance (or perceived arrogance) and it can be dangerous if the person concerned thinks they are immune to risk.

Hence the need to think before you speak when talking to your child. And of course, it all depends how you choose to bring them up. The opinion your child has of him- or herself will inevitably be influenced by your approach to child-rearing – whether permissive, authoritarian or liberal – while they are young; when they fly the nest they will come to see themselves as a person in their own right and become less influenced by other people's judgements. A child is a promise. And you must make sure that promise is kept by establishing a few principles that will give them good self-esteem, i.e. the right amount, neither too high nor too low.

For example, having clearly set up rules from the outset, make sure your child understands that failing to respect them will have consequences, which you must be careful to make proportionate. Force yourself, when possible, to give the child the opportunity to make his or her own choices. You may be dreaming of them becoming a goalie, but there is no point signing them up for the local football club if they prefer tennis. Or making them bash away at the piano if all their focus is on drawing. To coerce them is to undermine their assertiveness and that means undermining their future autonomy. To give them choices is to give them confidence.

It's important a child isn't restrained from expressing his or her emotions or opinions and that, whatever they choose to do, you offer encouragement and support to help them achieve the goal they've set themselves, using all the intellectual and material means that you can reasonably provide. By trying their best, they will bump up against reality, and failure or success too. But they will also learn a lot about what they are capable of and what they cannot do. This way, they will know themselves better. This way, they will accept themselves for who they are. This way, crucially, they will have the confidence to be open with other people and find their place, their own place, in a group or community.

Down with guilt!

Do you sometimes blame yourself? Regret not measuring up? Convince yourself you've done the wrong thing?

Yes? That means you are a prime candidate for three pieces of advice that will help you escape the guilt trap. It can wreak havoc, this trap, so you're well advised to keep it at a distance.

1. No one's perfect. Not even you. Not even me (not quite, anyway . . .). You have to convince yourself of that once and for all. It doesn't make you someone to steer clear of: quite the reverse. But accept it, convince yourself of it, and you will have

taken a massive stride towards improving your well-being. Recognizing one's faults and weaknesses is actually a calming thing.

2. The world is not black and white; it is grey. The colour analogy is intended to convince you that we all have a shadowy side. It makes us nuanced beings, and therefore worthy of other people's interest.

3. As children, we had a fairly binary view of the world. People said to us 'That's good' or 'That's bad' and we believed them. But aren't things a bit more complicated than that? The quest for perfection is bound to end in failure. Listen to your desires, your wishes, even if it means juggling with your scruples a bit (provided no one gets hurt). In a word, live!

The only thing worth beating yourself up about would be not finishing this book. But you seem to be on track. Well done. Keep going . . .

The importance of empathy

Well-being is also about your connection to other people. The way two people relate to each other, the clarity of communication between them, is what gives the phrase 'living together' its real meaning. In the sixties, the cry was: 'Make love, not war!' Today, we talk about empathy. And it's not just a buzzword: it's a formula to live by. Doesn't mean you shouldn't make love, by the way. But that's another story . . .

Anyway, back to empathy. Empathy means being capable of understanding someone else's emotions without any sense of judgement. Listening takes precedence. Interaction between you both must not be coloured by your own way of seeing the world.

So, be empathetic. It will do you as much good as it does the person on the receiving end, because you will need to be more open to others, develop your intuition and be tolerant of the fact that other people behave or think differently from you. Mind you, if you know you are a hypersensitive sort, be careful not to overdo the empathy, which can cause you to lose perspective and feel exactly what the other person is feeling. That is not the aim of the exercise. Being empathetic is like driving in traffic: you should always keep a safe distance from the car in front.

Don't confuse **empathy, sympathy and compassion**. Empathy is a subtle ability which enables you to understand someone's distress. It differs from sympathy, which is about feeling sadness for the other person ('I'm so sorry'), and compassion, which makes us share that person's suffering ('You're crying? I'm crying with you!'). After all, if we use these different words it's because they often express different meanings.

Pollen protection

Among the huge army of people with pollen allergies there are those who know it and those who don't. Yup, as strange as it sounds, some people aren't aware they are allergic to pollen. Which is why it's useful to keep an eye out for the symptoms.

A runny nose? Blocked nose? Could be rhinitis. Your eyes are watering? Itching too? Maybe it's conjunctivitis. Your throat feels blocked? Making a noise like a locomotive when you breathe? That sounds like asthma. *Atishoo!* Hay fever?

If that all sounds familiar, you're probably allergic to pollen. It usually starts in March with the arrival of spring and lasts until September. These symptoms can make your life a misery so it's not a bad idea to arm yourself with some strategies for reducing them. Here are five suggestions that can work alongside any medical treatment your doctor sees fit to give you:

1. Wash your hands, nose, face and eyes thoroughly and frequently.
2. Do some serious housework at home; dust more than usual.
3. In the car, drive with the windows up: keep that pollen on the outside!
4. Consider shielding your eyes with sunglasses, and maybe even wearing a protective mask. I can think of more glamorous accessories but at least it's effective.
5. If you spend some time in a garden or park during the day, wash your hair in the evening before going to bed. Like you, I prefer pollen to be down the plughole rather than on my pillow.

Look after your memory effortlessly

Have you ever had a memory lapse? Forgotten someone's name, where you put your keys, the right way to the right place? Of course you have. Because from day to day our memory has fun playing tricks on us. Memory, whether tactile, olfactory, auditory or visual, lets gaps appear. They needn't overly worry us or get us mumbling about Alzheimer's, but they remind us that our memory needs a certain amount of maintenance. It's like democracy or freedom of the press: if we don't use it, it erodes. Fades. Dies out. And that's a great pity, because Nature gives us memory so early in our existence, long before our birth apparently: most scientists agree that a foetus is able to remember smells, sensations, tastes and the sound of its mother's voice.

The seat of memory is the hippocampus, located in the medial temporal lobe beneath the cerebral cortex. Am I boring you? I know . . . I bore myself sometimes. Let's simplify things: the seat of memory is the brain . . . And do you know that the brain is 80 per cent water? So your memory is directly affected by a lack of water. Dehydration leads to problems with concentration, and concentration is what helps memory function properly. I'm sure you can deduce from this that drinking water regularly, without waiting to be thirsty, and eating foods that are rich in water, such as fruit and vegetables, are good ways to preserve your memory.

The brain also consumes a lot of oxygen: it alone soaks up 20 per cent of the oxygen we absorb. There is one way to ensure it's well oxygenated: exercise. We keep coming back to the same obvious answers, I know, but I believe there is a pedagogical virtue in saying the same thing over and over again. And, by the way, you'll find that repetition is your memory's best friend. Another thing: after a workout, the body releases endorphins, the hormones that encourage concentration, memory's other ally.

Things designed to make modern life easier are making us lose habits that are really useful for maintaining our memories. Rather than writing by hand, we tap on a keyboard. The good old notepad has been replaced by the screen. But writing longhand stimulates zones of the brain that relate to thought, language and memory. Don't completely shun two objects that are becoming more and more obsolete: a pen and paper. Nor should you yield entirely to the magic of the camera phone. We use it to snap away left, right and centre without realizing it's altering our ability to remember things properly. Researchers have identified what they call 'the depreciation effect', a phenomenon that comes about when we use cameras as a prop. Technology can certainly be a useful way to remember something or someone, but it mustn't stop you taking the time to look around you, which is one of the ways that we oil the cogs of our memory day to day.

And speaking of oil (bit of a kamikaze transition coming up), now seems a good moment to recommend olive oil to you. Not only does it have a direct impact on memory, but it is a key component of the Mediterranean diet, which is known to protect the brain from the effects of ageing.

The basic principles: eat nuts; choose fish over meat, for its high content of polyunsaturated fatty acids and its top-quality proteins (salmon, tuna, mackerel, herring, sardines); swap cows' milk for ewe or goat; and prioritize fruit and vegetables, which are high in minerals, fibre and antioxidants. The latter fight free radicals that love to go for poor defenceless neurons.

Antioxidants can be found in foods that are rich in vitamin C (red fruits, citrus fruits, Brussels sprouts, broccoli) and vitamin E (potatoes, pumpkin and sunflower seeds), as well as garlic, beetroot, carrots, mushrooms, lemons, spinach, kiwis and apples. To complete the shopping list, stock up on magnesium in green and leafy vegetables and dark chocolate. Magnesium has the distinctive feature of actually increasing our stock of synapses, the brain's nerve endings that transmit information, and this can only have a positive impact on our cognitive function.

As you can see, maintaining your memory is also about lifestyle. It all boils down to small behavioural choices that, over time, work towards keeping our long- and short-term memory systems intact. Don't feel guilty about giving in to a little nap.

That's good for the memory. A short sleep in the middle of the day helps us assimilate the information we took on board that morning. A scientific study has shown that cerebral activity is greater in someone who has napped than someone who hasn't.

Don't feel guilty about wanting to go for a stroll either. Artificial light is all very well but, even if yours is the most pleasant of offices, your body really needs natural light. Remember to get some of it in the middle of the day. By doing so, you will help synchronize your sleep and improve it for the night to come. Your memory will be strengthened too, because it's during deep sleep (the deeper the better) that your brain compartmentalizes all you have absorbed during the day.

On top of all these good habits, I could add the moderate consumption of coffee (caffeine stimulates the long-term memory and improves visual memory); the urge to laugh (when we laugh, the brain releases endorphins, the hormones that improve concentration); and reading. Reading improves your cognitive performance because it demands imagination, comprehension and memory. Basically, it gets the brain working.

Learning one or several **foreign languages** is very good for the memory. MRI scans carried out as part of a study on the subject found that people who speak at least two languages use their brain more efficiently and are also exposed to fewer memory problems than those who only specialize in English (being able to speak American too doesn't count!). In fact, as you might imagine, the more time you spend speaking other languages, the more you stimulate your memory. *Capito? Entendu? Verstanden? Comprendido?*

Short-term memory and long-term memory

The human memory is capable of storing billions of pieces of information in the brain. But I should say 'memories', plural, because we make a distinction between our short- and long-term memories.

The first has a reduced storage capacity, sometimes greatly reduced. It can have a lifespan of as little as 0.5–10 seconds. It still has a job to do, chiefly instructing our senses to filter elements for retention in the flood of information that our eyes, ears, fingers and nose capture. What is usually defined as short-term memory lasts about 30 seconds. This length of time allows us to retain information long enough to, for example, dial a phone number we have just been given or grab a pen to write it down. It is possible for us to extend the duration of this memory by repeating the information that needs retaining over and over again, in our heads or out loud. This type of memory is precious: it plays a central role in accomplishing daily tasks.

Within this short-term memory, psychologists have identified what they call the 'magic number seven'. We are thought to be able to retain, briefly, seven different units of information, either visual or auditory. But not everyone has signed up to the same tariff! Some people are limited to five, others can get up to nine. It all depends on the individual's capacity to concentrate. In any case, this series survives for about 20 seconds in our brain, on average. After that, 90 per cent of the information is lost. Along with the coachloads of useless information that is forgotten instantly, to save our brains from saturation.

The transition from short- to long-term memory occurs thanks to repetition or the power of emotion. This is what enables us to construct individual memories, a phenomenon explained by Hebb's Rule, named after the Canadian neuropsychologist Donald

Hebb (1904–85). When a neuron regularly sends a message to another neuron, the latter becomes increasingly sensitive to this message. A link is created that unites the two neurons and this link is strengthened if the connection is repeated, increasing the chances of that particular memory being maintained over time. This is how we remember our times tables or recitations. But emotions can produce the same effect. When the first neuron is activated by an image that is out of the ordinary, whether it relates to a happy event (a birth, for example) or some sort of violent act, say, the emotional charge instantly solidifies the memory. We sometimes say, 'That was unforgettable.' And we really mean it; we won't forget it. This event will be recorded in a durable way in the part of our memory that has an indefinite storage capacity, theoretically unlimited, called long-term memory.

This memory has a storage function and our personality is constructed around it. We have it to thank for the memories of our first holiday by the seaside, the way the sensation of our first kiss stayed with us, the fact we can recite a few lines of poetry or remember the rules of poker. It's this type of memory that enabled Proust to evoke the aroma of madeleine cakes dipped in herbal tea from his childhood, a princely use of olfactory memory. This is the strongest of the five senses, more evocative than auditory, visual, tactile or taste memories, thanks to specific neurons spread along the nasal cavity that are capable of recognizing 10,000 different smells.

Long-term memory comprises several processes: implicit memory, which subconsciously manages learning (how to walk, for example), and declarative conscious memory that manages acquired knowledge, which we can draw on when the need arises. However, we aren't all equal when it comes to the mechanisms of memory. Memories imprint themselves better before we reach 30, the age at which powers of concentration reach their height. After that, things drop off. A teenager can do his or her revision listening to music but someone in their forties would need silence. Around 50, the memory starts to feel its age and this process speeds up after 75.

But age isn't the only factor to consider. Sex (whether you're a man or a woman, not the practice . . .) can also have a say. For example, women are often iron deficient. Now, iron is vital for transporting oxygen to the brain, so a shortage of iron directly affects the ability to memorize and concentrate. That means it is in your interest, ladies, not to turn your noses up at a bit of black pudding, red meat, offal, lentils, spinach and wholemeal grains, all of which are bursting with iron.

Genes, upbringing and profession also determine our capacity to remember. People who have worked their memory throughout their life by intellectual activity, and built up a 'reserve' as a result, will have more chance of delaying the onset of problems. A Swedish study has shown that in a stimulated brain, even an older one, the neurons are renewed a lot more frequently than we once thought, at a rate of 2 per cent a year.

Fascinating memory! The Greeks were right to dedicate a goddess to it: Mnemosyne. (If you're wondering whether that's where the word 'mnemonic' comes from, the answer is yes.) Born to Gaia (the Earth) and Uranus (the Sky), Mnemosyne had a particular gift: she invented words and told stories. To charm Zeus, god of gods, she regaled him with tales of victories over their enemies, the Titans. Zeus succumbed and, on the summit of Mount Olympus, Mnemosyne gave birth to nine daughters: the Muses. The ancients sometimes painted her as quite a mature lady, supporting her chin in her hand and holding her ear lobe between the first two fingers of her right hand, to suggest reflection. This is something of an exception because it was more usual, in the Ancient World, to depict gods as young people. Perhaps it was a way of highlighting how important she must have been before the invention of the alphabet and writing. Unless it was an attempt to capture the precise moment that the two memories, short and long term, cross over; the precise moment the brain receives a piece of information, processes it, gives it meaning and decides to keep it. Or not.

We're forever bemoaning the fact our memory is going, but is it possible, conversely, to have too much memory? The answer is a resounding yes. This phenomenon has a name: **hypermnesia**. If I ask you where you were ten years ago on a certain day and at a certain time, what you were doing, with whom, having eaten what, and you are able to answer me in full, this may be cause for concern (don't panic: a one-off notable event can occasionally justify having a memory like an elephant). If, on top of this, you are prone to aggression, anxiety, paranoia, loss of libido and recurring nightmares, you should see a doctor because these are the symptoms of hypermnesia. It could have been brought on by a physical shock (as can amnesia) and it requires medication coupled with psychological aftercare.

Everyday memory

Along with my previous comments about how and why you need to maintain your memory, which does inevitably erode over time, there are hundreds of tricks to avoid short-lived and perfectly benign memory problems that are nevertheless annoying and waste time. I call these tricks 'instant memory'.

You will have heard of President Franklin Roosevelt. This former president was elected four times, a unique feat in the history of America. But that's not all he is known for: he had an exceptional memory. He had no trouble remembering the name of someone he had met only once before. So what was his secret? When confronted with a stranger, he visualized their name written across their forehead. You just have to remember to do it and devote 5 seconds or so to the exercise. First, it's useful to really look at the person as they tell you their name for the first time. Perhaps ask them to repeat it. Then repeat it yourself, to make sure you're got it right. Look at their face; match it to the name. In 15 seconds the information will be recorded in your memory. And, hey presto, you've done it.

Do you take notes during meetings or conferences? No? You should. Re-read them shortly afterwards, underlining the most salient points. Doing this little task will help you retain the elements that merit retention. Add diagrams and visual elements: images will help anchor knowledge in your memory, particularly if you have a visual memory.

Lost your keys? Put your glasses down somewhere? You call that looking? Have a proper search. Here's a serious suggestion: next time, talk to yourself. 'I'm putting my keys on the hall table.' Or, 'I'm putting my glasses in the top drawer of the desk.' Saying it in your head should be enough. But if need be, say it out loud. You will bring your auditory memory into play. Memory is organized in such a way that we remember things better if they are said to us. So, talk to yourself: it's better to *look* crazy than go crazy looking!

Can't find your car? Worried it's been stolen? Before you start falsely accusing people and calling the police, tell yourself it's a memory lapse. For the simple reason that you didn't get it working in the first place. Again, take a deep breath and repeat: 'I'm parking my car in front of the red gates' (although if the gates are blue, you might want to rethink the wording). Pausing for a moment once you've parked is another way of improving your chances of not losing the plot. Look around you, make a mental note of a few details such as the name of a shop, the colour of a shopfront or the name of the street. These observations will give you a mental snapshot of your location. When you return, the pieces of the jigsaw will surge forth from the depths of your memory as if by magic. Do only that.

There is no way you will remember anything while answering a phone call or having a chat about the latest must-see film. The key to memorizing is focus. If you're concentrating when you learn a new piece of information, you have a greater chance of retaining it than if you're in multitask mode, which happens too often in our super-connected society where we reply to text messages while doing something else entirely.

Is there a particular subject that fascinates you? Yes? Well then, you will have noticed it gets your memory working effortlessly. It's easier to remember things we're interested in, right? Numerous studies have shown that people who enjoy intellectual pursuits have better memories. Stimulation, learning and understanding make the cortex work and, as a happy side effect, keep our spirits up too.

Do you know your National Insurance number? No? It's quite handy. Why not learn it by heart, once and for all? Your ability to rapidly retain something like this will surprise you. Try learning a poem that made an impression on you, the words of a song you like humming, maybe even a few useful phone numbers (just in case you can't lay hands on memory's worst enemy, your mobile phone). These little exercises will stimulate your immediate memory. Repetition is the key to successful memorizing: it enables reliable connections to be made between the neurons.

Are you a procrastinator? Putting off until tomorrow what you would do today? If the answer is yes, try to kick this bad habit. Outstanding tasks block the memory. Free yours by doing things as soon as you think of them. It won't just be good for your memory, it will also be good for *you*, because procrastinators are usually self-blamers too. Another quirk of the procrastinator: once they have got going they want to accomplish *all* outstanding tasks. Mistake. They can easily end up intending to do one thing and actually doing another. They strive to do several things at once, too. Ever since the days of Aesop and his hare we've known that approach is doomed to failure. So, if you're easily distracted, choose to do one thing and stick with it. Ignore extraneous temptations that steer you from your first intention. Give it a go: it will do you good.

Do you work listening to music? It's not always a good idea. Some studies have shown it to have a distracting effect. It is said to reduce performance in terms of focus and memory. However, there is evidence to suggest listening to classical music prior to working is effective: it calms you down and improves concentration.

Take all these 'instant memory' tricks on board and the only risk you run is of being selected for the World Memory Championships. Yes, such a competition exists. It was created in 1991, takes place once a year and is getting more and more popular. Played out over ten disciplines including: memorizing a poem in 15 minutes; a number made up of dozens of digits in 30 minutes; as many faces and names as you can in 15 minutes; as many separate single numbers as you can in 5 minutes; as many random words as you can in 15 minutes; and as many historical dates as you can . . . Try remembering a sequence of 10 playing cards and you'll start to get an idea how hard it is. One person surpasses his peers at this game: the British man Dominic O'Brien. At the age of 58, he has won eight world titles. His most astounding performance? In 2002, he memorized a random sequence of 2,808 playing cards (54 packs), making only eight mistakes! I don't think I'll be challenging him to a game of blackjack . . .

Epilogue

I would like to end this book by quoting a man who revolutionized his own era and left a lasting influence on subsequent ones. That man is Henry Ford, the great American industrialist of the first half of the twentieth century. He once said of his success: 'If I had asked people what they wanted, they would have said faster horses.' And so, taking the opposite view from all his advisors, who were anxious to stick with what they knew and persevere with the horse-drawn carriage, he invented the Model T Ford. Its advent coincided with the spectacular rise of the automobile.

I like Henry Ford's phrase (the man himself wasn't without his faults, but that's another story) because it encourages us to raise the bar a notch, it invites us to make changes, it stimulates our capacity to 'Think different'. That, of course, is the slogan of another revolutionary business thought up by an undeniable visionary whose insight is still being felt today, the late Steve Jobs.

Nothing great, nothing lasting can be accomplished without an innovative approach and, when it comes to health, this lies within everyone's grasp. We can all innovate. If we really want to, we can resolve to change the way we live our lives. This ambition must be borne out every day in our actions, with good sense not guilt, with self-kindness not anxiety. You're a marksman in a shooting range, picking up his handgun and taking aim at a cardboard cut-out 25m away. If the barrel of the gun deviates by just a few millimetres, the bullet will finish up 2m from its target. The target is your well-being, your health and the pleasure you take from life. Those few precious millimetres are your capacity to adopt positive patterns of behaviour, to fight against all the bad habits that have won you over, some of which you may have recognized in these pages. So, aim well! Don't let the tip of the gun deviate from the right trajectory. Work to claw back each fraction of a millimetre, as represented by the chapters of this book. It exists to accompany you on your journey, long term.

I know your faults, they're mine too. This book is the friend who wants to see us succeed, the mate who knows us inside out, who puts an arm around our shoulders and explains that if we continue doing things the way we always have, we shouldn't be surprised if we keep getting the same outcome. You'll see, you'll get used to change more quickly than you think you will, because the way we live our lives becomes imprinted in our brains and produces lasting results. I'm telling you this because I'm convinced it's true, because I have experienced it for myself, because I have confidence in you.

With thanks to . . .

Sylvie Delassus, Capucine Ruat, Amélie Bastide, Isabelle Doumenc, Paul-Louis Belletante and Christophe Brun

Sources

e.sante.fr

Le Magazine de la santé, France 5

'The bio-business', Laurent Hakim and David da Meda, *Envoyé Spécial*, January 2012, France 2

'The false promises of *light* food', Laurent Dy and Lise Thomas-Richard, *Envoyé Special*, April 2015, France 2

Healing Without Freud or Prozac, David Servan-Schreiber, Réponses, Robert Laffont, 2003

Terra Eco

Allo-docteurs.fr

60 millions-mag.com (Institut National de la Consommation)

La Bio entre business et projet de société, under the direction of Philippe Baqué, Contre-Feux, Argone, 2012

'La qualité des produits de l'agriculture biologique et le PNNS', Denis Lairon, Inserm study

Inra.fr (Institut national de la recherché agronomique)

Journal of Agricultural and Food Chemistry

Ads you will never see again, Anne Pastor, Hugo Desinge, 2012–15